MAKING STUFF AND DOING THINGS

DIY Guides to Just About Everything
4th Edition

Edited by Kyle Bravo

Microcosm Publishing
Portland, OR

Making Stuff & Doing Things:
DIY Guides to Just About Everything

© Kyle Bravo, 2003, 2017, 2020
This Edition © Microcosm Publishing, 2003, 2017, 2020
Cover by Dan Cole

Major thanks to Jenny LeBlanc

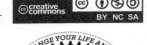

This is Microcosm #19
ISBN 978-1-62106-647-7

First edition (July 12, 2004) 3,000 copies
Second Edition (April 15, 2006) 6,000 copies
Third Edition (May 10, 2008) 8,000 copies
Fourth Edition (December 13, 2016) 5,000 copies
Fourth Edition, second printing (January 9, 2020) 3,000 copies

For a catalog, write or visit:
Microcosm Publishing
2752 N Williams Ave.
Portland, OR 97227
www.Microcosm.Pub
(503) 799-2698

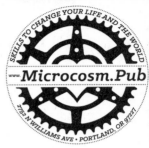

To join the ranks of high-class stores that feature Microcosm titles, talk to your local rep: In the U.S. **Como (Atlantic), Fujii (Midwest), Book Travelers West (Pacific), Turnaround in Europe, UTP/Manda in Canada, New South in Australia,** and **GPS in Asia, Africa, India, South America,** and other countries.

If you bought this on Amazon, I'm so sorry because you could have gotten it cheaper and supported a small, independent publisher at www.Microcosm.Pub

This book is for informational and entertainment purposes only. The content of this book is not guaranteed to be factual, scientifically valid, healthy, or safe. The reader assumes full responsibility for actions taken as a result of any article in this book and should take all possible safety precautions. Kyle Bravo, Microcosm Publishing, and the individual authors disclaim liability for any injury or damages resulting from the use (proper or otherwise) of any information in this book. Neither Kyle Bravo, Microcosm Publishing, nor the individual authors are responsible for the contents therein, the actions of readers in response to the articles contained in this book, or any consequences that may occur as a result of these actions. Breaking laws can have severe consequences.

While some of the contributors here directly or indirectly suggest minor property destruction like cutting locks on dumpsters or damaging compactors, the author feels uncomfortable advocating those kinds of actions and he would rather that you, the reader, consider choices that are right for you and focus on positive action instead of destruction.

Global labor conditions are bad, and our roots in industrial Cleveland in the 70s and 80s made us appreciate the need to treat workers right. Therefore, our books are MADE IN THE USA.

Microcosm Publishing is Portland's most diversified publishing house and distributor with a focus on the colorful, authentic, and empowering. Our books and zines have put your power in your hands since 1996, equipping readers to make positive changes in their lives and in the world around them. Microcosm emphasizes skill-building, showing hidden histories, and fostering creativity through challenging conventional publishing wisdom with books and booklettes about DIY skills, food, bicycling, gender, self-care, and social justice. What was once a distro and record label was started by Joe Biel in his bedroom and has become among the oldest independent publishing houses in Portland, OR. We are a politically moderate, centrist publisher in a world that has inched to the right for the past 80 years.

Library of Congress Cataloging-in-Publication Data

Names: Bravo, Kyle, editor.
Title: Making stuff and doing things : DIY guides to just about everything /
    edited by Kyle Bravo.
Description: 4th edition. | Portland, OR : Microcosm Publishing, [2016] |
    Graphical in nature, created in cut and paste style, or hand-written and
    drawn.
Identifiers: LCCN 2016014505 (print) | LCCN 2016023728 (ebook) | ISBN
    9781621066477 (pbk.) | ISBN 9781621069904 (epdf) | ISBN 9781621068884
    (epub) | ISBN 9781621068877 (mobi)
Subjects: LCSH: Handicraft--Pictorial works. | Do-it-yourself work--Pictorial
    works.
Classification: LCC TT145 .M3435 2016 (print) | LCC TT145 (ebook) | DDC
    745.5--dc23
LC record available at https://lccn.loc.gov/2016014505

CONTENTS!

- - - - - - -

FUN & ENTERTAINMENT

ARTS & CRAFTS

CLOTHING

CREATIVE TROUBLEMAKING

OUTDOOR SURVIVAL

GARDENING

FOOD & DRINK

TRAVEL

HEALTH AND BODY

PETS

REDUCE, REUSE, RECYCLE

REPAIRS

HOME SWEET HOME

TRANSPORTATION

INSPIRATION

FOLLOWED BY:

INTRODUCTION
TO THE FOURTH EDITION

When I reflect on how and why I came to compile a book about DIY, I have to go back to my teenage years. After a perfectly normal and comfortable childhood, in my teens came the explosion of "alternative" and "grunge" music into mainstream culture. I remember watching the "Smells Like Teen Spirit" video and just being blown away. All of a sudden I was exposed to a whole new world of weirdos and misfits that was intoxicating to a somewhat stifled and sheltered, middle class, suburban kid like me. It was through bands like Nirvana that I eventually discovered punk rock, through which I learned about the DIY ethic that underpinned much of punk culture, and it was that concept of DIY that became something of a guiding philosophy in my life for years to come.

My friends and I started a band. We wrote our own songs and then got a four-track and recorded them ourselves. We sat in our bedrooms and dubbed copies of our "album" on our stereos, cassette after cassette. We went to the copy shop and cut and pasted and photocopied our own covers. It was invigorating; enlivening; empowering. We had created something by ourselves, on our own terms, and it was awesome.

As I moved into early adulthood I was desperately seeking information and knowledge about other ways to live my life, to forge a path that was more authentically my own, making more intentional decisions about my day to day actions so that they more closely aligned with the ever-evolving ideals that were forming in my head and my heart. I sought out and soaked up everything I could, trying to learn how to make my life into what I wanted it to be. When I discovered the hidden yet vast subculture of self-publishing and zines, I became obsessed, reading and collecting every zine I could get my hands on, looking for whatever little kernels of wisdom there might be in those scrawled and photocopied pages.

The underground from which these zines emanated was teeming with a DIY spirit that was extremely attractive to me. I began collecting any and all DIY info that I came across in the zines I read. Anything I found that gave me clues toward living in a more real and intentional way, or that contained how-to advice or tips of any kind, made it into my ever-growing pile of photocopies. Eventually I had amassed quite a stack of articles on a wide range of subjects: gardening, cooking, fixing things, making stuff, doing things, etc. I decided to republish all of these articles in order to spread this amazing wealth of information and hopefully inspire a vast underground army of DIY pioneers who would take the ideas and put them into action. I put the articles together and published them as the *How2 Zine*. Many of the articles contained in this book came from this zine collection.

At the same time that I was working on the *How2 Zine*, a group of people at Tree of Knowledge Distro were putting together their own collection of DIY articles that they were hoping to publish in book form. Unfortunately, the Tree of Knowledge DIY book never came to completion, and though they had collected many submissions for inclusion in their book, none of them ever saw print. Eventually, thanks to the kindness and generosity of Tree of Knowledge, those submissions were passed on to me for inclusion in *Making Stuff and Doing Things*. I owe much thanks to Tree of Knowledge and, more specifically, John Gerken, for passing on so much great information.

This book is an amazing example of folk knowledge. The information contained in these articles is written, not by experts, but instead by ordinary, everyday people. The facts may not always be right, the science may not be exact, but the spirit is true and alive. Folk knowledge passes from person to person, from place to place, from generation to generation, and on through history in a way that no textbook could ever match. Sure it may be rough, poorly edited, even riddled with mistakes, but this is real knowledge about real people living real lives.

Looking back now I question some of my original decisions about which articles to include in the book because of the iffy advice that some of them contain or because they espouse certain actions that I personally don't agree with like property destruction. I want this book to be about taking positive actions to make ourselves part of a better world, not about negative or destructive acts, but ultimately we decided to keep all of the original articles in this edition to maintain the integrity of the original collection as it was when first published. Despite any flaws, this book is still a testament to the ingenuity and creativity of regular people.

Because of the long journey many of the articles in this book have taken—passing through many hands and much time—some of the original authors' names have been lost in the process. I made a significant effort to track down every author, but unfortunately not all of them were to be found. Also, because of the transient nature of the underground from which these articles came, many of the authors whose names were known were still unable to be located. I want to give credit where credit is due, so if you are aware of the author of an uncredited article, please get in touch. In the end, the decision was made to include certain articles even if their authors could not be found[1] because I felt that this book was about sharing knowledge and information that belonged to everyone, not restricting it.

When these articles were first written, the internet was in its infancy. Information was less readily available and connecting with other people who shared your weird and idiosyncratic interests wasn't as easy as just a few clicks of a mouse. Zines were a necessary and important medium for disparate seekers to connect to one another and create a space for themselves in the world, whereas today that space is found for many people online. Because of this, I think this book serves a different purpose today than it did when it was first published in 2004, functioning more as an artifact of a specific moment in time than a literal guidebook per se, though I do think the articles in this book still hold relevance now, some ten to twenty years after they were first written.

Ultimately, I hope that this book will find its way into the hands of a new generation, and that they will flip through its pages and discover a world of possibilities that they didn't even know they were looking for, and maybe at least a kernel of some kind of magic that simply can't be found online. If nothing else, I hope that this book stands for the idea that we don't have to just be passive consumers, but that instead we can take action to transform our world into whatever we want it to be, and that together, we can do it ourselves.

---

1 As the publisher of this book, Microcosm was only made aware that some of the articles had been printed without permission when their authors got in touch in late 2004. Otherwise, these articles would not have been included. We are very sorry to anyone whose work was used without their explicit permission and have since added safeguards as a result.

How to change the world in just four easy steps!

1. Get off yr ass.

2. Write, talk, listen, participate, read, volunteer, take in new ideas and spread yr own.

3. Repeat steps 1 and 2 many times.

4. Give another person these instructions.

Direct Action

Autonomy means direct action, not waiting for requests to pass through the "established channels" only to bog down in paperwork and endless negotiations. Establish your own channels. If you want hungry people to eat, don't just give money to some highhanded charity bureaucracy; find out where food is going to waste, collect it, and feed them. If you want affordable housing, don't try to get the town council to pass a bill—that will take years, while people sleep outside every night; take over abandoned buildings and share them, and organize groups to defend them when the thugs of the absentee landlords show up. If you want corporations to have less power, don't petition the politicians they bought to put limits on their own masters; find ways to work with others to simply take the power from them: don't buy their products, don't work for them, sabotage their billboards and buildings, prevent their meetings from taking place and their merchandise from being delivered. They use similar tactics to exert their power over you; it only looks valid because they bought the laws and social customs, too.

Don't wait for permission or organization from some outside authority, don't beg some higher power to organize your life for you. Act.

Do It Yourself
Do It Yourself OR DON'T

I've been thinking a lot about DIY projects and culture lately. It's really starting to pull together into a big picture and make sense to me. As long as I have been involved in this "punk" culture, I've been inundated with the idea of DO IT YOURSELF. And it makes sense that fixing your own bike will save you money, but I couldn't really see how these little things made that big of a difference. One of the things that frustrated me was that it is difficult to "do it yourself" when you don't know how and there is no one to teach you. So I started a little DIY website, which was quickly co-opted by Misterridiculous.com. Although I'm not a huge fan of the internet as a source of information (because it's kind of exclusive to those who have computer access and often information is incomplete and incorrect,) it was one way I could pass along what I know, and help others pass along what they know. Then I heard about the DIY skillshare in Bezerkely, CA and I was really inspired. I started reading <u>Taking Charge of Our Lives</u> by the American Friends Service Committee, and there was a lot of talk about community. They talked about having community shops and toolsharing, and really just working with each other. All this other stuff I've been reading, like Luddite Tech Zine, Seedhead and How 2 zine, have really started me thinking about how it can all be connected. Because the more we network, the more we can really step away from consumer culture. I figure the more that I can do for myself, the more I can do for someone else too. I can fix bikes, someone else can garden, or plumb or build stuff. Maybe I can do all that stuff anyway, but this person is willing to help me out if I'll help them out with their bike. I keep reading more about these communities that are becoming more self sufficient, and not having to rely upon grocery and department store chains, and that's where I really see the benefit in DIY.

Eight Things You Can Do To Get Active

1. Pay attention to where and how you spend your money. Is your money going to support companies that don't care about you? Are they destroying the environment, killing animals, treating your friends who work for them like shit? Are they trying as hard as they can to sell you a product that gives you cancer? Are their advertisements designed to manipulate you, to make you feel insecure or make their product seem like more than it really is? You don't need to give those motherfuckers your money! For that matter--do you buy many things that you don't need? Soft drinks and junk food at convenience stores, for example? Do you end up spending a lot of money whenever you want to relax and have a good time? There are a thousand things you and your friends can do that are fun, creative, and don't cost anything (having intense discussions, exploring hidden parts of your town, making music-- instead of drinking at bars or going to movies and restaurants) just as there a thousand ways you can eat and live more cheaply (Food Not Bombs, building furniture instead of buying it, living in big houses with a bunch of friends). Once you experiment a bit, you'll probably find that you enjoy life a lot more when you're not always shelling out cash for it.

2. Now that you spend less, you can work less, too! Think about how much more time that gives you to do other things. Not only will it be easier to do things that help you spend less, like volunteering at Food Not Bombs (the less you work, the more time you have to make sure you don't need to), you'll also be able to do all the things you never had time for before: you can travel, exercise, spend more time with your friends and lovers. When it's sunny and beautiful outside, you can go out and enjoy it!

3. And you'll have time to do the other things you need to do to take back control of your life and your world. First, start reading. It doesn't really matter what, so long as it makes you think about things and gives you new ideas of your own. Read novels about human beings struggling against their society, like J.D. Salinger's Catcher in the Rye or George Orwell's 1984 or Joseph Heller's Catch 22; read the beautiful, dreamers' prose of Jeanette Winterson or Henry Miller. Read history: learn about the Spanish revolution in the 1930's, where whole cities were run by the people who lived in them, rather than by governments; learn about the labor union struggle in the USA, or the Free Speech Movement in Berkeley in the 1960's. Read philosophy, read about environmental issues, read vegan cookbooks and underground 'zines and comics and everything you can get your hands on. Here's a hint: if there's a university in your town, you can probably get a membership for about $10 a year-- and most libraries include videos, too!

4. Reading isn't the only way you can expand your horizons and clarify your ideas. Talk to people about the things that interest you, arguing when you don't agree, so you'll get to know your own beliefs better. Write to the people who are doing the 'zines you like, discuss and debate things with them, ask them for directions to find out more about your interests. Try writing about your own ideas, and sharing that with people, until you feel confident doing this. Travel to different places, try to learn about other cultures and communities, so you'll have more than one perspective on the world and you can start to imagine what the world is like through other people's eyes.

5. Now you'll know what you want, and you can go about getting it. Seek out other people and groups with similar goals, and figure out how to support them or participate in what they're doing. Maybe

you can copy fliers and give them out at shows; maybe you can organize benefit shows for organizations you want to support (women's shelters, radical bookshops, local groups protesting against the execution of Mumia Abu-Jamal or lobbying for protection of the environment). Maybe there are public protests and demonstrations going on that you want to be part of. Try to help find ways to make these more challenging and fun than just a bunch of people holding signs; everyone's so bored with doing that that there must be a more effective and exciting way to go about it.

6. You can start your own projects, as well, you know. If there's no Food Not Bombs in your area, get a group of people together and find some local businesses that will donate their leftover food. If there's something fucked up at your high school or college or workplace, try organizing a walkout to force the "authorities" to do something about it... and to show everyone that those "authorities" only have as much power as we let them have. If the main street of your town lacks life and excitement, try organizing an unexpected festival to take place in the middle of it one weekend. Shake up everyone's lives and expectations, shake them out of their apathy and boredom so they'll start thinking about things. Establish networks with other people who are also interested in having an effect on the world around them, so you can help each other do this.

7. Through all of this, don't stop questioning yourself and your assumptions. Try to see through all the social programming you've received throughout your life: consider how gender roles constrain the way you act, how your own relationships with people reproduce the same hierarchical order that your fighting in mainstream society. We're not going to really change anything unless we can create new ways of living and interacting, new values that show themselves in the way we treat each other. Show your friends how much you care about them. Consider doing things you never thought you should or could do: dancing, singing, admitting things that you've been taught to be ashamed of.

8. Now look to the future. How can you stay involved with these things as you get older? How can you construct your life so you will always be free to do what you want to? Talk to people older than you who haven't given up and gone back to the daily grind of eat-work-sleep-watch TV. With a little input from them and a lot of resolve on your part, you can maintain your activities and your lifestyle as long as you want to. Idealism, adventure, and resistance don't have to be reserved for youth alone. History is filled with men and women who refused to compromise or calm down, who went all out from the cradle to the grave. They are the artists, the leaders, the heroes and heroines even people from the mainstream respect. We can all have lives like theirs, if we're brave and idealistic enough.

If all of us demand control over what we do and what goes on around us, if all of us do what we can to make life exciting and fair for everyone, things are bound to change. A lot of people know that we don't live in the best of all possible worlds, but persuade themselves that it's hopeless to try to improve things because they're afraid to commit themselves, to take any risks. But it's that lack of ambition that is the biggest risk of all--for what if you do nothing, and nothing happens, and we lose our chance to make this world the paradise it should be? Don't be shy or timid--there's nothing more exciting than taking an active role in the world around you, and there's nothing more worthwhile!

this message brought to you by the CrimethInc. Special Forces c/o C.W.C., 2695 Rangewood Drive, Atlanta, GA 30345 USA

Learning in Freedom- For Free!

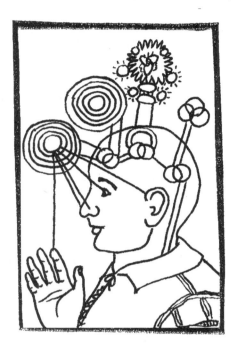

In America we are only expected to dedicate 13 years to education, perhaps with an additional 2-8 years for the particularly (and typically) ambitious and privileged. After that we are supposed to have all the knowledge we need, at which point we kick in into production mode of working to pay the bills. Not only is the idea that we have all the knowledge we need in this comparatively short period of time illogical considering the constant change and progress of the world around us, but it keeps us bound in production mode. The fact is, while the world is constantly changing, so are the people. They need more information not only to function in their jobs, but to satisfy the self--the part of us that is constantly changing, growing, evolving.

While we continue to learn through life experience, seldom do adults actively pursue education. Most people are content to come home from work, kick their feet up, and watch the television. There is no denying the fact that there are people that are just too exhausted after a day of working to consider getting out of the house in the quest for new knowledge. But how many of those people are watching the television out of boredom, loneliness, or because they simply think there is nothing better to do? Perhaps most people are responding to the cultural expectation that education is unnecessary after high school or college. It seems that the popular view point is that if learning isn't rewarded with a degree or a promotion, than it holds no value.

People who are living intellectually stimulating lives are obviously going to be a happier bunch of people, not to mention they are likely to posses superior critical skills and be able to identify more options/alternatives to their current way of living/working/communicating/creating/existing. Yes, what I am trying to say is that people actively pursuing knowledge are going to be empowered people. That is the reward, that is the end result.

Unschooling is often applied as a way of guiding children through their primary learning opportunities, but it does not have to be a way of teaching and learning that is exclusive to children. I don't know how many people have said to me, "I wish my parents would have raised me in a homeschool/unschool environment." Well, what is stopping them from unschooling their way through life, starting right now? Unschooling is not some magical idea floating on cotton candy clouds and sprinkled with fairy dust that disappears at puberty or when a person turns 18 or gets a full time job and rent payments.

To unschool as an adult (or teenager), I think three important things need to happen:

1. A commitment must be made. This means a faithful resolution to actively pursue knowledge regularly.
2. A hard step in the process: Throw away all pressures (from inside and out) that says learning must show profitable results or be rewarded with a degree or some other recognition. Learn simply to satisfy a need to know.
3. Begin actively pursuing the information and/or skills you want or need.

So that sounds pretty logical and simple. I'm guessing what throws people off the path is #3 on the list. Time, money, and resources get thrown into the mix and the whole idea begins to resemble the impossible. Sadly, we don't live in my imaginary utopian world where Free Universities exist in every town. As far as time goes, I wish I had some to spare. Do what you can. Squeeze in a class, read a book, or take a trip when you can find the time, wherever you find it. As far as money goes, I don't have any of that to spare, either, but I do have some practical ideas on how to get information and skills for free or at very little cost.

Free College Classes: If you would like to take a class at a local college but don't have the cash (and aren't trying to get a degree), you may be able to attend classes for no money. Write or e-mail (phone calls are probably a bad idea for too many reasons to list) the instructor teaching the class(es) you want to take and ask if you can sit in. Explain that you don't have the money to pay for the class, but that you have an earnest desire to learn, and they will likely let you sit in on their classes. This probably won't work for lab type courses where you would work with school supplied equipment, but most classes are lecture type settings, so sitting in should not be a problem. If one instructor turns you down, look for someone else teaching the class, look for other classes altogether that interest you, or look at a different school. Be persistent. It never hurts to ask.

Start a Learning/Teaching Collective: You would be amazed at how
many professionals are willing to talk about or demonstrate what
they do for free or for a small fee. Of course, most people aren't
going to want to come to your house and make a presentation to you
alone, but you get a group of people together and they will
probably do it. So you start a Learning/Teaching collective.
Begin by talking to some like minded friends about your idea, and
then begin to flyer and spread the word about what you are doing.
Give your collective a name, write up a mission statement and then
start organizing classes. You can hold meetings/classes in
someone's living room, a public park, ask the library to lend you a
conference room, or charge a small fee for each class to cover the
cost of renting a space.
Have an open meeting for generating ideas for classes/presentations
they would like to participate in. Here's a few ideas for
classes/people to contact:

*park rangers for environmental/ecology presentations
*photographers who can give photography/dark room instruction
*chefs, nutritionists or dieticians could teach vegetarian, ethnic,
pastry, or other cooking styles
*mechanics who can show how to change oil and present other basic
car maintenance techniques
*musicians willing to give an introductory course
*martial arts or yoga instructors willing to host a demonstration

The possibilities are endless. Start flipping through the phone
book and you are bound to come up with countless ideas.

Then assign willing members of the collective to call up
professionals and ask if they would give a free class/presentation.
If the group really wants to learn a particular thing but no one is
willing to do it for free, find out how much they will charge for
their time and then charge participants a fee (preregistration is a
good idea) to cover the cost. When talking to professionals, you
might want to drop a hint at what great advertising this could be
for their business. This is especially true for businesses that
teach classes already, like karate or something. Giving a free
class could boost their enrollment.

Be sure to flyer for all collective meetings and classes to
encourage others to participate. Another idea is to generate a
small free or low cost newsletter put out by the collective. This
is a way to advertise events, and it helps show potential free
teachers that their time and energy will be spent on a focused and
organized group of people. Perhaps the newsletter could also
include reports from classes/presentations, editorials, artwork,
and all kinds of other things that the whole collective can
participate in working on, which could turn out to be a great
teaching/learning tool in itself.

Book Discussion Clubs: A few pitfalls of being in charge of your
own education is that often you will find yourself without company.
Exchanging thoughts and ideas with others is not only a great way
to learn, it is also very motivating. Starting a Book Discussion
Group is one way to open up communication with people. Check your
local public and college libraries about existing book groups. If
there aren't any, or none that exist appeal to you, start your own.
Pick a focus for your Book Club. Maybe Science Fiction, Women's

Studies, Anarchism, French Revolution era literature, etc. Tell all your friends about the Book Club, put up invitations at local public and college libraries, book stores, and coffee shops. Set a date, time and location for the initial meeting. You can have it in someone's living room, a coffee shop, or ask the public library to let you use a conference room.

At the first meeting, have everyone submit ideas for books to read. You can vote on which book to read first, or throw all the ideas in a hat and pick one. Then decide what kind of time frame everyone wants to set for each book and then schedule the date, time, and place for regular meetings.

Apprenticeships: This one is pretty straight forward. If you know somebody that does something you would like to learn, just ask them to be your mentor. As long as you're not getting in their way, most people would be flattered by such a request. If you want to learn something and don't know anyone who does it, drag out that phone book and start making calls. Ask to observe someone while they are working at what they do; tell them that you are very interested in the kind of work they do and that you would like to get an up close look.

It may feel a little awkward asking someone to mentor you at first, but just remember that up until recent history, apprenticeships were the way that most skills and arts were taught and passed along through the generations. In many parts of the world this kind of teaching/learning is still how most people learn their trades. And the fact is, there are plenty of obscure (for one reason or another) arts and skills that aren't easily learned by reading books alone. If you are interested in something, seek out people who are doing it and form a relationship with them in some way with the obvious intent of furthering your education, plain and simple. Trade Unions are something to look into if you want to learn a skill that will include a job in the learning process. Each Trade Union has different stipulations about how to join and other matters like apprenticeships, so your best bet is to call the local Union Hall of the trade you are interested in and ask a lot of questions.

Libraries: This one is pretty obvious, isn't it? The library is just full of all kinds of resources. Not only can you get books about every subject under the sun and use the internet for free, but most libraries hold regular cultural arts presentations. So drop by there regularly and pick up a schedule of events and an armload of books.

Booklist

What follows is a list of books that may be of interest to those curious about Homeschooling and Unschooling. This list is in no way complete -- there are many sources of information out there on a wide variety of topics that tie into the subject. The books below are most useful to those who are exploring the possibilities -- they deal more with philosophy and technique than curriculum and technicalities. I've tried to divide the titles into three distinct categories in order to make it easier to locate the appropriate source for particular information, but please keep in mind that in one way or another all of these books are related and compliment each other well.

Critiques of public school and prevalent education techniques:

Lessons From The Mississippi Freedom Schools*
By Kathy Emery & Linda Gold (eds)
Gives a history of the Mississippi Freedom Schools, curriculum information and discusses education as an act of civil disobedience and social change.

A Different Kind Of Teacher: Reflections On The Bitter Lessons Of American Schooling*
By John Taylor Gatto
A critique of the American public school system with possible strategies to create change.

Deschooling Our Lives*
By Matt Hern (ed)
Offers a critique of the current American school system and offers education alternatives by way of Home, neighborhood and communtity based education.

Talking Schools*
By Colin Ward
Ten lectures from a Libertarian perspective regarding education and public schools with possible solutions to percieved problems.

Dumbing Us Down : The Hidden Curriculum of Compulsory Schooling
By John Taylor Gatto
A popular critique of the American public school system.

Homeschooling:

Freedom Challenge: African American Homeschoolers*
By Grace Llewllyn
A collection of essays of special interest to African families interested in home based education.

And the Skylark Sings with Me - Adventures in Homeschooling and Community-Based Education
By David H. Albert
A personal account of one family's experience with Homeschooling.

Allison's Story : A Book About Homeschooling (Meeting the Challenge)
By Jon Lurie, Rebecca Dallinger (Photographer)
A photo journal of an 8 year old girl's experience with Homeschooling. A good way to introduce young children to the possibility of home education.

And What About College? : How Homeschooling Can Lead to Admissions to the Best Colleges & Universities
By Cafi Cohen, Patrick Farenga (Editor)
Helpful to teenager's in a Homeschool setting, as well as parents concerned about Homeschooling's impact on the future of their young children.

Real Lives: Eleven Teenagers Who Don't Go To School*
By Grace Llewellyn
An excellent companion to the previous book.

Learning All the Time
By John Caldwell Holt
Considered the grand-daddy of the Unschooling movement, this book
explores the philosophy of Unschooling in depth.

Charlotte Mason's Original Homeschooling Series
By Charlotte Mason
This is the complete works of the turn-of-the-century British
educator, Charlotte Mason, who is considered the pioneer of
homeschooling. Includes theory about child behavior and
development and parenting.

Family Matters : Why Homeschooling Makes Sense
By David Guterson
Written by a former English teacher and novelist (Snow Falling
onCedars) who homeschools his children. Covers many aspects of
Homeschooling with a fluid writing style, of course.

Unschooling:

The Unschooling Handbook : How to Use the Whole World As Your
Child's Classroom
By Mary Griffith
One of the most mainstream and popular books about Unschooling.

The Teenage Liberation Handbook: How To Quit School And Get A Real
Life And Education*
By Grace Llewellyn
An essential for teenager's and parents alike. Explains the
philosophy of Unschooling, legal aspects, dealing with parents,
curriculum possibilities and more.

* These books are available at www.akpress.org or write for a
caralog:
AK Press Distribution
674-A 23rd Street
Oakland, CA 94612
USA
Please support independent writers, publishers and vendors-
especially if they are radical!

Of all the books I have read on the subjects of homeschooling
and unschooling, I was most inspired by Grace Llewellyn's books
on unschooling. On the last page is a order form to get
them direct from the publisher. If you are considering buying a
gift for a young person, please give them one of these books. I
really believe these books have the potential to help people
change their lives.

Kevin taught me how to write.
Not by teaching me grammar or sentence structure.
But by telling me that he's a writer
and that I am too whether I admit it or not.

Ward taught me how to sing.
Not by teaching me scales and octaves.
But by telling me to be loud and to be brave.
To sing loud and out of tune is to sing
nonetheless.

I'm teaching myself how to draw.
Not by taking classes or lessons.
But by filling empty pages with ink blotches and
scribbles.
By taking the time to give myself the chance.

Dan taught me how to swing an axe.
He showed me the grip and the stance.
He told me not to stress over it,
to let the axe do the work.
Then he let me swing it all day letting
me do the work it took to figure it out.

Good teachers are ones who know when to stand
aside and let people use the skills they were
taught and their own knowledge to figure things
out. Too many times we see failure in trial-and-
error. We give up on ourselves as teachers and
students.

-To my friends, the great teachers
   in and out of classrooms.

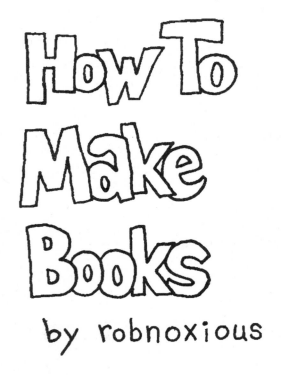

How To Make Books

by robnoxious

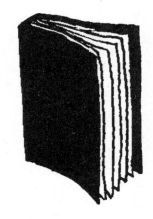

During the last months of 1999 I was trying to figure out how to publish the counterculture novel I had written. I was broke and no good at saving money. I got tired of waiting around for a rich relative to die. I considered applying for a grant, but instead managed to convince my partner to loan me a thousand bucks. I called around and got quotes from printers and bookmakers. I considered all kinds of things until I settled on printing up the pages at a web printer (on newsprint), then trimming the pages myself and binding them into a cover that I would print the artwork on by hand. I decided to make the books myself because it cut the cost in half, and half of the cost was all the money I had! All I had to find was a printer to print the actual pages and then I could do the rest of the work.

When I first thought of making my own books I thought it would be too hard and take too long. I discovered that it's not so hard to make a decent little paperback book with a cardstock cover. If the only popcorn you know how to make is microwave popcorn, and the only other food you eat is from the drive thru at the local fast food can, making books is not for you. It takes a little time to figure it out at first, but hopefully this article will send you in the right direction.

First, what's the difference between a DIY zine and a DIY book? Well, same ethics, but a book is a one shot deal with no issue numbers. The disadvantage is that every time you go to distribute it, nobody has ever heard of it, so you don't have that name recognition like zines that have a hundred issues out. But I think making a book also has a few advantages. There's no real limit on size. You can make a book as thick as you want whereas saddle stapled zines have a definite limit on how many pages you can fold and staple. Also, a book has at least a cardstock cover that makes it more durable and permanent. I like that a lot. By making a book I'm creating something that people can keep and pass on because it doesn't decay as fast as zines do. I like the idea that I'm not fueling the consumerist urge. The longer my publications last, the longer our wounded forests can last too.

I wanted to make my own books because I could reuse cardstock that had been discarded into recycling bins at photocopy stores. Not only was that free material for the covers, but it also saved the value of the cardstock before it was destroyed and made into toilet paper (every time paper is recycled the fibers are weakened so that it can't be made into the same thing, but only something weaker).

I also liked the idea that the creation of the book did not end when I wrote it, but flowed all the way through until I physically handed the thing to someone and completed the circle. I think the message from this act is just as strong as the written messages in the book – that the medium you use is the message. The message that a handmade book gives is not of factories and consumerist plastic perfection, but of a feeling, imperfect, passionate human being behind the creation.

For about $700 I got 2000 copies of my book printed onto good quality newsprint. That makes each book less than 50 cents to print. I just called around asking for price quotes from web printers. Usually in bigger cities you will find better prices. I printed my book at a place in North St. Paul called Lillie Suburban Newspapers. There was also another place with a good deal that would have printed 5000 copies of my book for about $1400. Once a printer has everything set up it doesn't cost much extra to print a few thousand more.

Another method is offset printing – a high quality printing method usually done with regular white paper. It's a lot more expensive, even if you can find a supportive printer that gives you a good deal. I did a book years ago that was offset printed by some punks in Berkley and cost $1800 for 1000 copies. They looked nice – they were perfect, but I now prefer a lesser quality so that I can have more books at a cheaper cover price. The offset books cost $1.80 each to make whereas the newsprint ones cost about 60 cents each including printing the covers, etc, but not including my per hour labor for binding which I decided not to charge myself for.

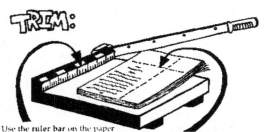

Use the ruler bar on the paper cutter when trimming the card stock covers. When you know the exact length and width you can line it up to those measurements and trim them easy.

Mark the **trim lines** on your master copy before you send it to the printer, that makes it easy to line up the printed books on the paper cutter!

Whatever type of printer you decide to use, make sure you communicate with them, and aren't afraid to ask questions if you don't understand or else your misunderstanding will be multiplied a thousand times over! One of the most important things is to use the right size fonts because some will be too small to be legible when printing with newsprint. Get a sample of things the printer had made before to give you an example of how things will look when printed. Also, if you have a book with pictures or words that you think might be offensive to the printer you might want to sit down with them first and straight up talk to them about it. This is much better than letting them get into the job and then decide they're going to fuck with you for the content of your book.

Once I got all the folded newsprint books back to my attic I figured out how to trim them on my paper cutter. The easiest way is to figure out how you will cut the things before you send them to the printer and draw little marks or lines where there needs to be a cut. The paper cutter I got was about $50, but it can only cut through half the thickness of my book. It would be nice to use an industrial cutter so that I would only have to make four cuts, but they cost more than a thousand bucks, so, instead, I make eight cuts on my cheap trimmer.

There are many artistic methods you can use to put an image on the cover of your book. Stickers and stamps are easy methods. You could even have a stamp made by professional stamp makers for pretty cheap. Linoleum block cuts also work good. Once, for the covers on a full size zine, I stuck my hand flat onto a plate of black paint and pushed my palm down onto the front cover – a human stamp!

On my newsprint book I'm using a silkscreen to put the image on the cardstock covers. It's the same sort of silkscreen that puts images onto t-shirts. This is a whole other DIY process which is covered elsewhere in this book. Books on silkscreening are also easy to find at the library.

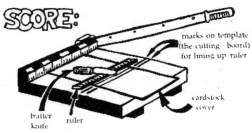

marks on template (the cutting board) for lining up ruler

cardstock cover

butter knife

ruler

First, I cut the cardstock to the right size for the cover, then screened the image onto the cardstock, then let it dry. I had a thick string with a bunch of clothes hanging pins on it that I clipped the cover up on to dry. If I didn't hang up the covers, then Yoda, our cat, would have added her artistic touch by walking all over them. When the covers were dry, I did the scoring which made the two folds for the spine of the book. To score, first make a template. I used the surface of the cutting board because it has lines already and an edge to butt up against. Measure on the template where the folds are, then make two marks with a permanent marker. Put a ruler lined up on the marks and then hold the ruler down with one hand and run a butter knife along the straight edge. If you end up with two pieces of cardstock, you need a duller knife. You might want to run the knife more than once, or push harder, depending on the thickness of your cardstock. Now fold the cover along the two lines you just scored.

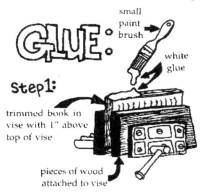

small paint brush

white glue

Step1:

trimmed book in vise with 1″ above top of vise

pieces of wood attached to vise

The way I decided to bind the books was with water-soluble white glue like Elmer's. It stays pretty flexible when it dries which is important for a book. I also got a very small paintbrush to brush the glue onto the spine of the pages.

I got a very cheap wood worker's vise ($10) and attached two flat pieces of wood slightly larger than the book so the entire book could be held in the vise. I took the trimmed book and racked it down on the table to make sure all the pages were down by the spine side. Holding it tight, I put it into the vise and closed the vise. I left about an inch of the book sticking out the top of the vise. I then took the brush, loaded it up with glue, spread a good amount on the even pages of the spine, making sure to get them all. A good bead of glue is ideal. I took my fingers and wiped alongside the book. If there is glue on the outside of these pages it will squish up and glue the outside pages to the cover!

I then racked the book down on the table, spine side down, to seat the pages in the cover. Then I put the book, spine side down, between two heavy objects so that it remained upright while it dried overnight.

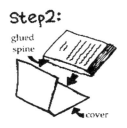

Step2:

glued spine

cover

An alternate way to bind books is by sewing the spine. I do this sometimes when I have a cardstock that is glossy on the inside because the glue will not stick to it (reused cardstock such as cereal boxes, etc.). For this type of binding, rather than trimming the spine of the pages, I instead fold the pages like a regular zine with a saddle fold. You need a needle and thick thread or dental floss (which I prefer) and a thimble to push it through. I put the book on top of a folded bath towel then put the pages and the cover together. Next, I stabbed the needle through from the inside fold of the book, pulled it through to the outside, then stuck it back through. I then cut the floss, tied it up good, and pulled the knot tight.

If there are single pages that are not connected in the saddle you can also stab sew through the side of them. Just put them in the cover and stab away. Stab sewing is tricky, but it's probably more permanent than glue, and it's also vegan (many glues have animal parts in them).

When the book was dry the next day, I took both sides of the cover and opened the book. I turned it upside down and jiggled it. If any pages fell out, I glued them back in individually. If enough glue was put on while the book is in the vise and it's worked in good with the brush, this hardly ever happened.

If you follow these steps you will have created something unique with your energy and spirit. This is an excellent project for someone who is quitting or cutting down on smoking, drinking, taking drugs, etc. It gives you plenty to do with your hands and your time. Why just sit around listening to records when you can make the words in those lyrics come alive in your hands? Success is not out of reach. Make a new definition of your own life. You could convince some friends to help you with it, or do a joint book project, or a compilation, so they all could share in the work of creation.

WHY MAKE A ZINE OR ARTIST BOOK?
→ SELF - EXPRESSION! ←

- **ZINES** ARE A FUN WAY TO GET YOUR ART (& ETC.) "OUT THERE" WITHOUT WAITING FOR "PERMISSION" FROM ANYONE! NO EDITORS TO PLEASE, NO ADVERTISERS TO WORRY ABOUT OFFENDING, NO WAITING!! TRUE UN-CENSORED, NON-COMERCIAL FREE SPEECH!

- **ARTIST BOOKS** ARE WORKS OF ART THAT CHALLENGE ARTISTS TO THINK IN BOTH 2D AND 3D! ARTIST BOOKS OFTEN BECOME ART OBJECTS AKIN TO SCULPTURE! FINE ART THAT IS INTIMATE LIKE A GOOD BOOK! COOL!

* LIBRARIES COLLECT ZINES AND ARTIST BOOKS! *
A LIST OF LIBRARIES AND OTHER WONDERFULNESS CAN BE HAD
FOR A DOLLAR FROM: ZINE LIBRARIAN ZINE
P.O. BOX 12409
PORTLAND OREGON 97212

STARTING...

- FIRST THINK OF A TOPIC YOU WANT TO MAKE A ZINE/BOOK ABOUT.
- SKETCH OUT A LAYOUT/FLOW OF HOW YOU WANT YOUR "STORY" TO GO, WHAT YOU WANT TO SAY. A "STORY" DOESN'T HAVE TO USE WORDS! (PAGES TURN IN A RHYTHM OR FLOW)
- MAKE A BOOK "DUMMY" — THIS LETS YOU EXPERIENCE THE SIZE AND BINDING TYPE THAT'LL SUPPORT YOUR "STORY". IT ALSO LETS YOU DOUBLE CHECK YOUR PHYSICAL STORY FLOW.

* THERE ARE MANY WONDERFUL BINDING TYPES FOR BOOKS BUT FOR THIS ZINE WE'LL DISCUSS THE MOST BASIC CODEX FORM! WE'LL CREATE A SINGLE SECTION CODEX

CODEX – PAPER SHEETS, FOLIOS OR SECTIONS ARE ATTACHED ALONG ONE EDGE – CREATING A SPINE

CODEX BOOK

(CODEX BOOK TYPES MAY HAVE MANY SECTIONS)

PAGES IN A SINGLE SECTION OR "PAMPHLET"

MAKING PAGES (SECTIONS, ALSO CALLED SIGNATURES)

WE'LL USE 8.5 X 11 SIZE PAPER FOR OUR PROJECTS BUT THE CONCEPTS APPLY TO ANY SIZE PAPER.

Ⓐ SECTION TYPE ONE (FOLIO)

A FOLIO IS A SINGLE SHEET FOLDED IN HALF (EITHER LANDSCAPE OR PORTRAIT) WHICH MAKES 4 PAGES. TWO OR MORE 8.5 X 11 FOLIOS ASSEMBLED TOGETHER BECOME A SECTION. (MAKES A 5.5 X 8.5 SIZE FINAL BOOK OR 4.25 X 11 SIZE BOOK)

INPOSITION IS HOW PAGES ARE PRINTED OR DESIGNED SO THAT THEY ARE IN THE CORRECT ORDER.

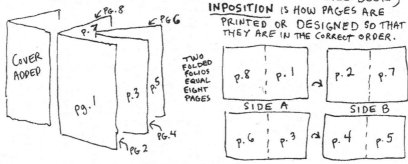

Ⓑ SECTION TYPE TWO (QUARTO)

OR YOU CAN MAKE A QUARTO. IN A QUARTO THE SINGLE FOLDED FOLIO IS FOLDED YET AGAIN TO CREATE MORE PAGES OUT OF A SINGE SHEET. (8 PAGES FROM ONE SHEET) YOU'LL WANT TO FOLD THE PAPER AND NUMBER THE PAGES AS WELL AS MARK THE HEAD OR TOP OF EACH PAGE TO HELP ORGANIZATION. (MORE SHEETS CAN BE FOLDED SIMILARLY FOR MORE PAGES, JUST ADJUST THE PAGE NUMBERING AS NEEDED. COVERS & END PAGES CAN BE ADDED AROUND THE FOLDED AND ASSEMBLED SECTION)

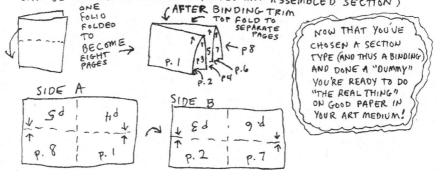

NOW THAT YOU'VE CHOSEN A SECTION TYPE (AND THUS A BINDING) AND DONE A "DUMMY" YOU'RE READY TO DO "THE REAL THING" ON GOOD PAPER IN YOUR ART MEDIUM!

BINDING

AFTER DESIGNING AND CREATING ALL OF YOUR PAGES, MAKE
THE COVER AND ENDPAGES (IF DESIRED). THEN MAKE ANY
DESIRED MULTIPLES (FLAT UN-BOUND PAGES XEROX EASIER).
AND YOU'RE READY TO BIND THE COVER, END PAGES AND SECTIONS.
→ NOTE: CROCHET THREAD WORKS WELL, AS DOES EMBROIDERY FLOSS
    BUT OF COURSE LINEN OR COTTON BOOKBINDERS THREAD IS BEST! ←

(A) 3-HOLE PAMPHLET STITCH ✳ (USE A TAPESTRY NEEDLE!)

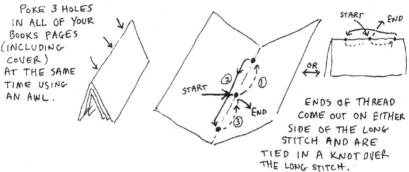

POKE 3 HOLES
IN ALL OF YOUR
BOOKS PAGES
(INCLUDING
COVER)
AT THE SAME
TIME USING
AN AWL.

ENDS OF THREAD
COME OUT ON EITHER
SIDE OF THE LONG
STITCH AND ARE
TIED IN A KNOT OVER
THE LONG STITCH.

(B) 5-HOLE PAMPHLET STITCH

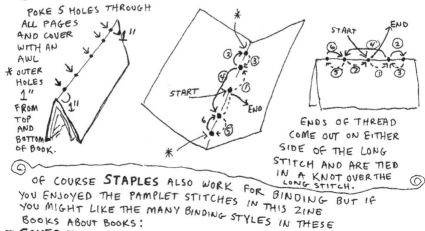

POKE 5 HOLES THROUGH
ALL PAGES
AND COVER
WITH AN
AWL
✳ OUTER
HOLES
1"
FROM
TOP
AND
BOTTOM
OF BOOK.

ENDS OF THREAD
COME OUT ON EITHER
SIDE OF THE LONG
STITCH AND ARE TIED
IN A KNOT OVER THE
LONG STITCH.

OF COURSE **STAPLES** ALSO WORK FOR BINDING BUT IF
YOU ENJOYED THE PAMPLET STITCHES IN THIS ZINE
YOU MIGHT LIKE THE MANY BINDING STYLES IN THESE
BOOKS ABOUT BOOKS:
- **COVER TO COVER** BY SHEREEN LA PLANTZ
- **MAKING JOURNALS BY HAND** BY JASON THOMPSON
- **NON-ADHESIVE BINDING VOL.1** BY KEITH A. SMITH

How To Make Your Own Movies
Mark Myers

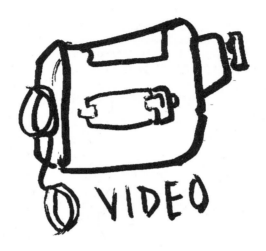

Every year we are bombarded with what seems to be an endless amount of mass-produced, multi-million dollar films that result in high ticket prices and bored, worn out minds. Instead of letting ourselves be victims to these corporate giants, we can learn to be our own best entertainment. How, you might ask? Simple. With a video camera, a few friends, and a creative mind, your own ideas can be put to video, giving movies the originality and entertainment qualities they were meant to have.

A video camera is probably one of your greatest (and most expensive) necessities in moviemaking. Though, there is no need to go out and spend a large sum of money on a camera. More than likely, someone that you know already owns one that sits in a closet, gathering dust, awaiting the next family event. If not, newspapers and ad bulletins have many inexpensive used cameras for sale. Always keep in mind that more money spent does not necessarily mean better quality.

Any amount of people can be used to make your movie – even as few as one. Yes, that's right, you can make an entire movie all by yourself. It all depends on your specific idea.

One movie that a friend and I made consisted of us switching off the acting and the videoing amongst those involved. This gave us more characters to work with in our storyline. Though, this only works if you keep at least one character off screen at all times in every scene.

Sometimes the hardest part in making a movie is coming up with the plot and storyline. Most people feel that they have to write out a screenplay with all the lines and actions of the characters. This is fine to do, though very time consuming and not always necessary. All of the movies that I have worked on have consisted of a small idea that we would build on. The idea would be given to the actors who would then act out the scenes and create the dialogue on the spot, with the scenes ending (shutting off the camera) when a prefigured action/word is done or said. Often the story and ideas grow while making your movie as you and those you are videoing get into the roles of the characters and your ideas feed off each other.

Movie costumes and props can be found in almost any home, closet, garage, refrigerator, etc. Some objects that seem so goofy and fake can look amazingly real on tape. Always be creative and open-minded for everything you find to use. Sitting around the house is an added movie prop that you do not have to buy. There is no better feeling than making a really good short movie without spending a dollar.

If you are videoing without a preplanned script you pretty much have to video the scenes in sequence. Working in sequence helps out a lot because it calls for less editing, if any at all. As far as editing goes, many people think that you need fancy machines. But that's bullshit; all you really need is a television, VCR, camera (or a second VCR, if available), CD/tape deck (for added soundtrack), and a lot of tv/stereo cable. I can't remember the exact hook up that was used by my friend and I, but the try and fail, try and prosper method always works with just about anything as long as you remain persistent. Just be patient and you will probably figure out something that works.

Finally, when making your movie, always remember these three basic necessities: creativity, originality, and patience. All three are greatly needed because no matter how short or inexpensive the movie you create, like any other form of art, you must feel its passion and drive. Otherwise you will just be wasting your time.

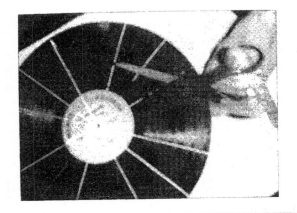

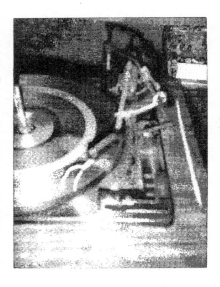

RECORD RECYCLE REUSE REPAIR

NEW USES FOR OLD VINYL

The following activities can be performed at home, in school, at work, or abroad.
Recommended for ages 6 & up.

BY The MONGER, as told to John Pugh x1.00

"I can only say that I am astonished and somewhat terrified...
astonished at the wonderful power developed--and terrified
at the thought that so much hideous and bad music may be put on
record forever."

--Sir Arthur Sullivan
1888

The world is overflowing with shit. Waste of every kind flows through
our homes at a steady rate;matching that of our consumption and sub-
sequent defecation.We eat food and drink liquid so that we can survive,but apart from that our waste is pleasure-based. We like to have
"things" that give us pleasure or comfort or convenience.It is a
trait we share as humans.However our appetite is massive and our tastes
fickle.Wegorge ourselves on "things" only to puke or shit them back.
out when we are finished.This is where waste comes from:leftovers,
regurgitation,packaging,refuse,etc.Space is limited on this tiny planet,so we either bury the waste where noone can smell it or we convert it
it into something useful--recycle it.Perhaps in its new form the waste
will find a purpose previously unconsidered.Perhaps its purpose will slo
slow the tide of shit that crowds our homes,our minds,our buttholes....

In other words,it's time to convert shit into gold.

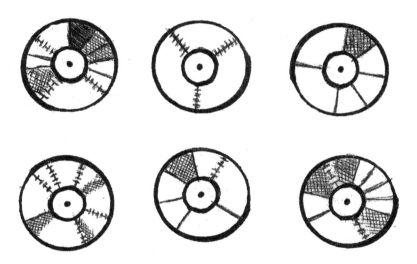

The diagrams are blueprints for beats that can be easily built
and played using any vinyl record (12" LP recommended) and a pair
of ordinary household scissors. A ruler and a white out pen can
be used to bisect and mark the exact degrees. A solid line indicates a deep rut should be carved into the surface f the vinyl.
A dotted line indicates a cut with scissors. A shaded area indicates
a series of close cross-hatches with the blade of your choice.
All these beats are just ones I figured out and can be fucked with.
Hours of fun are to be had around the old gramophones listening to
those beats battle it out.We recommend clearing the room of extran
eous furniture and invite over the neighborhood.

3rd Sleeper denies any responsibility for damaged needles or stereo
equipment that may suffer at the mercy of these
homemade beat records. You have been warned.We recommend trying out
some of our homemade amplification devices. Read on...

I.THE LISTENING CONE

This is the most basic and in some ways the "original" method
of stereophonic amplication. The idea came to us via Mr Wizard's
World. It is a simple idea that can be assembled at home using
household items. If you have to,consider this a science experi
ment for school.
Materials
One large(12"-24") piece of posterboard or construction paper
One medium sheet of aluminum foil
One safety pin or needle or paper clip
Tape (duct or masking)

1.Form the poster board into a cone.(The larger the cone,the
  louder the sound).Tape it in place along the seam.
2.Mold the aluminum foil around the tip of the cone.
3.Insert the needle or pin into the tip of the aluminum.
  Tape it if necessary.
4.Spin the record on a turntable or any concentrically rotating
  plane and apply the listening cone to the surface.

POSTER BOARD   TAPE

TIN FOIL
DIAPHRAGM

Safety Pin
NEEDLE

II.THE AMPLIPHONE

Here is where [___] Third Sleeper found volume.This still is
Primitive,caveman-level technology,but is often successful
in translating beats at a new threshold. This can also can
be assembled at home, but requires the sacrifice of an
otherwise "functioning" appliance.

Materials
One pair of headphones (preferably the large pre-90s model
  with $\frac{1}{4}$" jacks)
One safety pin
Tape (duct recommended)

1.Remove one speaker from the headphones.It should run direct
to the jack.
2.Strip the headphone of its cover so that the inner cone paper
  is exposed.
3.Straighten the safety pin so that it lies flat.
4.Puncture the inner cone paper with the safety pin;from the
  back,out through the front.
5.Tape the pin in place so that the sharp end protrudes at an
  angle at least an inch from the surface of the speaker.
6.Apply the device to the record while it is plugged into
an amplifier/stereo.The speaker translates as a microphone.The
  pin should rub up against the inner cone paper as it traces
  the topography of the vinyl surface.

NOTE:I run into limits with this device.
The weak ampliphone tends to feed back
easily when pushed to a significant volume.
Some folks like feedback.But it prevents
practical use outside of recording processes.
In a live setting,it is unpredictable,but in
recording it can be played "as loud as humanly
possible"The ampliphone operates best as a handheld
device,though it can be afixed to the turntable in a number of positions.

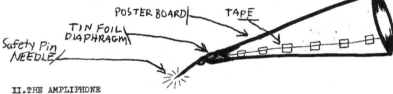

III.THE FANG JOCKEY

The Fang Jockey is a simple device of pure brute force. While it lacks the ability to translate musical notes from the record or follow the path of the predetermined grooves, it has proven to be very durable,withstanding a considerable amount of abuse and manual manipulation.The Fang tends to accentuate the surface per cussion of the vinyl while retaining a distinct bass bump and high smack.Once again the sacrifice of a semi-working apploance is necessary.It is bloody work this...

Materials
One turntable sans needle   cartridge
One paper clip
Tape(optional)
1.Remove the needle cartridge from the tone arm.If you look
  at the underside of the arm you should see a felt rubber
pad or hoop.This is your diaphragm.
2.Bend the paper clip so that it is nearly flat.Allow a slight
  bend so that the tip protrudes at an angle.
3.Insert the butt end of the paper clip in the end of the tone arm.
  If you can,loop it through the diaphram or puncture the diaphram
  so that the paper clip will rub up against it.
4.Tape the clip in place if necessary.Sometimes it will hold by
  itself.

NOTE:In order for the Fang Jockey to work
at maximum capacity,tinkering is always a
must.Make sure the paper clip is positioned
so that it does not tear the diaphram.
Since the Fang Jockey rides the vinyl in a
bareback fashion, it is sometimes necessary
to put a leash on the beast.A piece of wire
wrapped around the tone arm and anchored to
arm stand keeps the Fang bumping on a particular

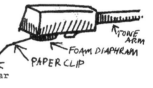

TONE ARM
FOAM DIAPHRAM
PAPER CLIP

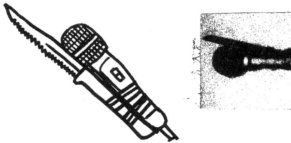

IV.The KnIFE MIC

This one should be pretty self-explanatory,but I'll break it down
for you...
Materials
One knife (preferably a sharp-tipped cutting knife no
  bigger than a bread knife)
One microphone(preferably a round-headed mic)
Tape(duct recommended)

1.Tape knife to mic so that the blade touches the mic's head.
2.Plug into a very loud amp and apply knife to turntable.

v.DOUBLE FANG ✶

Again this should be obvious having read number III,but
I'll be blatant...
Follow instructions forIII only form paper clip so that both
ends extend from tone arm.

✶ PICTURED ON TITLE PAGE.

EIGHT TRACK LOOPS

There is a flood of unused,unwanted,broken,warped,essentially
useless(but far from extinct)music committed to the format of
8-Track cartridge. The 8-track is designed to play in an album
long loop.Instead of two sides such as those on vinyl and cassette
tape,the 8-track is broken into four programs.Usually each program
includes 3 or 4 ssongs(and even at times half songs that continue
on the next program).The programs switch both automatically and
manually.At the conclusion of the fourth program the series repeats
itself starting at program one.   If left to its own devices
the cartridges will play infinitely.Keeping this in mind,a simple
loop can be put together with a little dissection.

1.Crack open the casing of the cartridge by
  pushing in the three plastic tabs indicated
  You might have to just break the tabs and
pry open the cartridge with a blade;just as long
as you dont severely damage the infrastructure
of the cartridge casing.

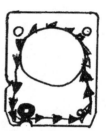

2.Remove the guts(reams of magnetic tape)but keep
  all other bits and pieces(felt pads plastics
  etc.)in place.

3.Cut a section of the tape approximately the
  length of the circumferance of the tape's path thr
  through the cartridge.Tape the two ends together
  in a hoop.Make sure the shiny dark side is on
  the outside of the hoops and the paler opaque side
  is on the in-side.However if you reverse this
  the loops will simply play backwards,which can be
  be just as rewarding.

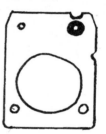

4.Place the tape loop back into the cartridge,follow
  ing the inner path as indicated.Replace cartridge
  casing,taping it in place if necessary.

5.Plug into any 8-track player.It will not damage
  the player in any way.Though the tape may come
apart if not properly assembled.You now have four
completely random loops appproximately 7-8 seconds in
length each.Press the program button to move from
loop to loop.

AUDIO CASSETTE LOOPS

This method of loop-building is similar(nearly identical)
to the method employed with 8-tracks so I wont spend much
time on it.The same process of dissection and removal of
guts is followed.We recommend you find a tape case assembled with screws so that you can take it apart and reassemble
with ease.The tension of the tape may take some serious trial
and error but the end result is almost always nastay!

COMPACT DISCS

Third Sleeper has found these new-fangled CDs to be adaptable
to our caveman mentality.Slight incisions made with a blunt rock   PICTURE
across the label surface(not the shiny side)cause malfunctions
that produce facinating albeit unpredictable results.This is   NOT
a delicate operation and could easily result in complete silence
if operated on without finesse.Play the mutilated CD in a regular   AVAILABLE
player(though some weaker ones may not co-operate).You made need
to push it along with the skip/scan button;be patient.This laser
technology is extremely volatile.

REEL TO REEL LOOPS

These loops are in some ways the most ideal.The tape can be any
length,but must be fed through the mechanism by hand.Remove
the plastic reels for easy manuver through the inner heads.
The speed of the tape loop can be manipulated by controlling
the tautness with the fingers.

HOW TO PLAY GUITAR

PLAYING GUITAR REALLY ISN'T THAT HARD. I SUPPOSE IT
MAY BE KIND OF FRUSTRATING & AWKWARD AT FIRST
BUT, JUST LIKE ANYTHING ELSE, THE MORE YOU
PRACTICE THE MORE IT STARTS TO COME NATURALLY.
YOU DON'T HAVE TO BE A GUITAR WIZ WITH EXTENSIVE
KNOWLEDGE OF MUSIC THEORY, OR SCALES, OR
CHORD PROGRESSIONS, OR ANY OTHER TECHNICAL
MUMBO JUMBO TO PLAY GOOD MUSIC. ALL YOU
REALLY NEED IS A LITTLE BASIC KNOWLEDGE
& A LITTLE INSPIRATION. HERE'S A FEW BASIC
THINGS TO GET YOU WELL ON YOUR WAY TO
BEING A TOTAL ROCK STAR!

TUNING

BEFORE YOU CAN PLAY YOUR GUITAR IT NEEDS
TO BE IN TUNE. FOR THE MOMENT WE'LL JUST
FORGET ABOUT CRAZY BANDS LIKE SONIC YOUTH
WHO LIKE TO TUNE THEIR GUITARS IN CRAZY
UNUSUAL WAYS, AND WE'LL JUST STICK TO THE BASIC
NORMAL WAY TO TUNE. SO HERE'S YOUR GUITAR:

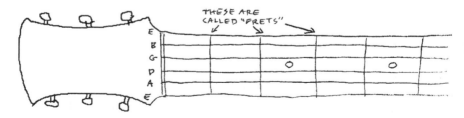

THESE ARE
CALLED "FRETS"

E
B
G
D
A
E

WHEN YOU'RE HOLDING THE GUITAR & LOOKING DOWN
AT IT THE LOWEST PITCHED STRING IS THE "E"
STRING, IT'S THE ONE CLOSEST TO YOU. NEXT
IS THE "A" STRING.

THEN COMES "D" THEN "G" THEN "B" THEN "E" AGAIN. THE LAST STRING IS AN "E" TOO! OK, SO HERE'S WHAT YOU WANT TO DO TO TUNE. PLACE ONE FINGER JUST IN FRONT OF THE 5th FRET ON THE LOWEST "E" STRING (AGAIN, THAT'S THE ONE CLOSEST TO YOU).

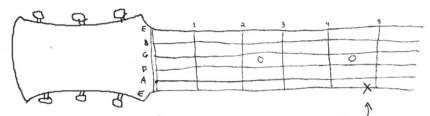

WHILE PUTTING PRESSURE RIGHT THERE PLUCK THE STRING & LISTEN TO THE SOUND it MAKES. NOW, ALSO PLUCK THE "A" STRING TOO. NOW IF YOUR GUITAR IS IN TUNE THEN THE OPEN "A" STRING & THE 5TH FRET OF THE "E" STRING SHOULD SOUND THE SAME. IF THEY DON'T THEN YOU NEED TO MAKE SOME ADJUSTMENTS. YOU'LL NEED TURN ON THIS TO ADJUST THE PITCH HIGHER OR LOWER TO MAKE IT INTUNE.

SO, ONCE THOSE TWO STRINGS ARE IN TUNE WITH EACH OTHER JUST MOVE ON UP TO THE NEXT STRINGS AND DO THE SAME THING. THIS IS HOW YOU TUNE ALL THE STRINGS EXCEPT FOR ONE. WHEN YOU GET TO THE "G" STRING (NO, NOT IN YOUR PANTS!) RATHER THAN HOLDING DOWN THE STRING ON THE 5TH FRET, YOU HOLD DOWN THE 4TH FRET. SEE THE DIAGRAM AT THE TOP OF THE NEXT PAGE.

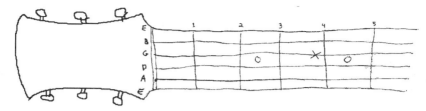

ALRIGHT! SO NOW YOUR GUITAR IS IN TUNE. NEXT WE'LL LEARN TO PLAY CHORDS!

CHORDS

THESE ARE JUST A FEW OF THE MORE BASIC CHORDS. IF YOU LEARN THESE AND CAN GET COMFORTABLE PLAYING THEM & SWITCHING FROM ONE CHORD TO THE NEXT FAIRLY QUICKLY THEN YOU'LL BE TOTALLY SET TO ROCK! HERE'S HOW IT WORKS: JUST LIKE THE TUNING DIAGRAMS, WHEREVER THERE'S AN "X" THAT'S A SPOT THAT NEEDS TO BE HELD DOWN. FIGURE OUT WHAT'S MOST COMFORTABLE FOR YOU AS FAR AS WHICH FINGERS YOU PUT WHERE. EVERYONE DOES THINGS A LITTLE DIFFERENTLY. ALSO, KEEP IN MIND THAT THE POSITIONS YOUR FINGERS HAVE TO BE IN TO PLAY SOME OF THESE CHORDS IS REALLY AWKWARD AT FIRST. BUT AS I SAID EARLIER, THE MORE YOU DO IT, THE MORE NATURALLY IT WILL COME.

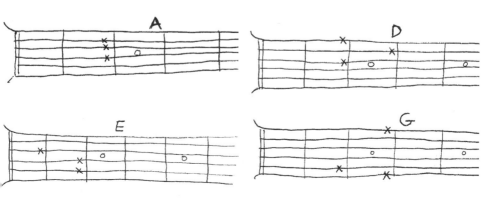

HOW TO JUGGLE

2 BALLS

I learned to juggle 2 balls before I learned 3 balls, but I've heard from others that it's easier to learn 3 balls first. Do whatever seems easiest to you. Basically all you do to juggle 2 balls is hold them both in one hand. Then throw one up in the air. Once it gets to the top of its arc throw the other ball up and get ready to catch the first ball. Pretty much as soon as you catch it you're gonna need to toss it up again because before you know it the other ball is gonna come right back down. This can be kind of frustrating at first, but trust me, the more you do it, the more you'll get used to the way it works, and soon enough it will be second nature to you.

3 BALLS

Juggling 3 balls is a bit more complicated to explain but I'll give it my best shot. Start off with 2 balls in one hand & one ball in the other. Throw one ball into the air out of the 2-ball hand.

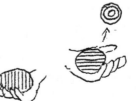

you want it to travel in an arc over to the opposite hand. When the ball gets to the top of the arc you need to throw the ball in the hand it's headed to into the air in a similar arc-like fashion. This will free up that hand so that you can catch the first ball you threw up. But get ready because now you've got another ball in the air about to come down! So, once again, when that ball is at the top of its arc, throw up the other ball. And you just keep going and going like that. Now go show all your friends how cool you are.

Hey, here's an exercise you can do at first that will help you kind of get used to how it feels to juggle 3 balls. Get just 2 balls and hold one in each hand. Throw one ball up in an arc, when its at its peak throw the other ball up in an arc then catch the first ball. Now catch the 2nd ball in the other hand. TADA! You did it! Do that a bunch of times. It should help.

OF COURSE YOU DON'T HAVE TO GO OUT AND SPEND TONS OF MONEY ON FANCY JUGGLING BALLS. YOU CAN USE ANYTHING — TENNIS BALLS, ROCKS, FRUIT, WHATEVER! OR YOU COULD EVEN **MAKE YOUR OWN JUGGLING BALLS.** HERE'S HOW:

Get some 9" balloons, and some bird seed or dry sand, or something like that.

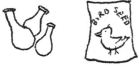

Fill up a balloon with whatever filling you're using. You're gonna need to really force it in there, so get a marker or a stick or something and use it to shove that stuff down in there. Once you get the balloon filled to a size you like you need to cut off the neck. Now grab another balloon and cut off its neck too. Take this balloon & stretch it over the stuffed balloon. Try to position the two openings on opposite ends, that way the filling won't come out. You might want to put another balloon layer or two on to make your balls more sturdy and long-lasting. And there you have it. DIY juggling balls!

A MAGIC TRICK

I'VE BEEN WANTING TO LEARN HOW TO DO MAGIC TRICKS LATELY. HERE'S ONE I LEARNED THAT'S EASY

YOU WILL NEED! A PENCIL · A PIECE OF PAPER · SOME TAPE

1. Cut off a piece of paper that's the same length as the shaft & roll it into a tube around the pencil & tape it.

2. Now, if your piece of paper is white, then it will appear that you have a white pencil. Say something like "Observe! In my hand I hold a white pencil!"

3. Now wrap the pencil in a piece of paper and leave just the eraser tip sticking out. Say something like "Abracadabra!" then tell someone to pull the pencil out of the roll of paper.

4. Oh my goodness! The pencil has magically turned from white to yellow! (assuming that it was a yellow pencil to begin with)

5. Gracefully bow as you are showered with applause.

Book Binding for Beginners...

There's a ton of variations on how to make your own book, but this is just one way, my basic recipe. Once you start you'll figure out other ways of doing it.

Decide how many pages you want total and in each signature. A signature is just a few pages sewn together. I usually use 3-4 pieces to a signature. Now fold the pages in half and stack them together. For example, if you want a book using 30 pieces of paper and have 10 signatures do this:

(3 pages folded in 1/2 for each one)

line them up and make marks with pencil where you will sew them.

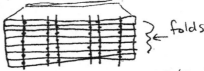

← folds

Use a ruler if you want the pages to be more exact. and do an even number of hole marks. now you gotta sew each signature to one another. i use dental floss, but any thread is good; waxed is just stronger. Start with a long piece. Also, poke holes with a needle into all those holes. Now you can sew. You can sew each one seperate and then sew them all together, or connect them all from the beginning. i find it easiest to sew them seperate first if the book is big. that way the sew job will be tighter by the end. Smaller books i usually connect the stitch. i'll demonstrate both ways.

Seperate:

tie a knot on the outside. leave a long end for tying. Thread the paper through each piece as demonstrated. tie tightly and knot the outside (also leaving another long end.) do this to each signature. then put all them together in a stack and tie the ends to one another tightly. Then sew the other signatures together any which way, as strong as you can, so they all tie together.

OR ... the interlocking method is basically to keep the pages sewn to one another at the same time that you sew the signatures together. Also, keep tying knots at the end of the pages. keep it really tight the entire time. First, get to the end of the 1st signature, and go into the 1st hole of the second. then, go into #2 from the inside, and loop around the string joining the 2nd + 3rd holes from the 1st signature. then go into hole #3 of the 2nd signature. keep going and do the same on the next holes. Basically, it's just making the 2 signatures joined. when you get to the end, tie a knot and start on the third signature. Remember to keep interlocking the signatures and tying the ends. after you've done, it'll look like this:

(You gotta do it, it sounds confusing but it's not once you do it!)

Remember to tie knots and it'll all be good and strong. When your thread runs out, just tie a knot + keep going!

Now you've got a book! Well, almost... you just need a cover. 1st, get some glue and run it on the spine, getting it in good and all over. Then put a piece of fabric around it, like so:

a little bit over on the top and bottom. make it tight. the key to a well bound book is over all tightness in the whole process.

Now, get materials for a spine and both covers. Cardboard is good. You want to cut out pieces only slightly larger than the paper or it'll get bent (unless you use a strong material... experiment.) but the spine should be the same size. Find some fabric, or like tubes joined together, or whatever, and glue them to the cardboard. leave some room between each piece for movement. Like so...

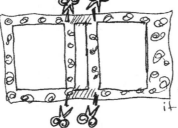

leave like ½ or ¼ inch between each and about ½ inch on all sides. Next make cuts on all sides where i marked. Fold down the fabric over and glue it to the spine part.

next, place your book inside, matching up the spines. Don't glue the spine down. take the first page of the book and glue it to the cover cardboard. do the same on the back. Then glue the cloth edges over the piece of paper. (or under — your preference)

SILK SCREENING!!!

EQUIPMENT: frame, silk, photoemulsion, sensitizer, squeegee,
(available at most art & craft supply stores)   ink, 100 watt light

1. Get an IMAGE, and copy it onto a TRANSPARENCY.

2. Get a FRAME

   and stretch the silk onto it.

3. Mix up 4 parts PHOTO EMULSION to 1 part SENSITIZER.
   (approx. 5 tsp. will cover an 8½"x 11" screen)

4. Spread an even layer on screen and lay FLAT to dry in a
   dark closet or other place completely void of light.

5. Once dry lay the transparency flat & BACKWARDS on TOP of
   the screen.

6. Place a light source with a 100 WATT BULB
   about 1 foot directly above the screen, allow
   it to be exposed for approx. 1 HOUR.

7. Spray the screen with a strong stream of water until the areas of the
   screen that were not exposed to light have washed away.

8. Once the screen is dry place a dab of ink INSIDE the frame
   and SQUEEGEE it across the image area.

9. Lift up the screen and BEHOLD your
   REALLY COOL freshly printed image.

Making Rubber Stamps

By Matte Resist

Making rubber stamps is incredibly easy. I can usually throw something simple together in about 5 minutes. All you need is:

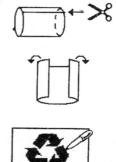

- An old inner tube (like from a bicycle)
- A scissors (or very sharp knife)
- Rubber Cement
- Something to glue your stamp to (like a block of wood)

First thing is to cut a piece of tube long enough to put your design on. Then cut it down one of the ridges so you can lay it flat. Brush off the powdery substance on the inside, and draw your design (on the smooth interior of the tube.. this way your design will look nicer. If you use the outside, the design will have lines running through it and rough areas) with a permanent marker. It will be difficult to see, but I can't think of anything else that would work better (and not harm the stamp).

Next, use a scissors to cut out your design. You can try to use a sharp knife, but this is difficult because of the way the rubber stretches. I've found a sharp scissors to be much easier.

Once you're satisfied with your design, find something to glue it to. A block of wood about the same size as the design is good. Otherwise, any flat surface will do. I've used the bottom of a whiteout bottle, the bottom of a tape dispenser, even an old CD.

For larger stamps if you can get your hands on a piece of foam about 1/16 of an inch thick, that will make things a look a bit nicer. Smear rubber cement on your block of wood (or whatever) and then on a piece of foam the same size as your wood block. Let them dry, then press them together. Then do the same with you're the design you've cut out. Smear cement on the rubber & on the foam, let them dry and then press together. (this will give you a much more solid hold than if you just apply the rubber cement wet and stick them together wet)

If you've used foam, using a sharp knife, cut the foam around the outside of the design, about as close as you can get to the rubber. Then peel the extra foam away This will make it so that when you apply the rubber stamp, you won't end up with the edges of the woodblock.

Then, just push the thing into an ink pad and apply to whatever.

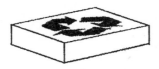 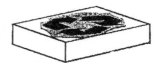

Block Printing- The Very Basics

This article was graciously done by Less, formerly of "to avoid suffocation."

Materials you will need

(you should be able to find these at most art supply stores)
Exacto Knife
Wood or Mounted linoleum
Speedball Carving Handle and Gouges sizes 1,2 and 5
Ink or think acrylic paint
Roller- called a brayer- soft rubber
Wooden or plastic mixing Spoon

There are 4 basic steps to the printing process **designing, transferring, carving and printing.**

The first thing to do when **designing** the image for your block is tint the surface of your linoleum. I use a broad tipped permanent marker in red or green. Color the entire top of the block an even shade of the color. Next draw an image that you would like to print on a sheet of paper the same size as the block. Draw this in pencil be sure that your lines are heavy and dark. This helps in the transfer of the image to the block. For your first attempt, choose a simple two-toned image with good contrast between light and dark. Also, if you are attempting text, remember that you have to carve it backwards if you want it to print the right way.

To **transfer** the image turn your drawing upside down onto the block. Lightly tape the image down. Use the mixing spoon to rub the back of the paper, use gentle yet firm circular strokes. After you have rubbed the entire sheet peel up a corner to check if the image has transferred well. If so peel off the paper, if not go back and rerub the places that haven't until you are satisfied with the transfer. Go over your pencil lines with a permanent black marker. Mark off all of the areas that you want to print in black so that you don't accidentally cut them out.

The next step is to **cut** away all of the areas that are not black, leaving a raised surface that will accept the ink and print onto the paper -- just like a rubber stamp. I start with an exacto blade and trace all of the lines with a shallow cut. I then follow with a number 1 speedball blade that I also outline all of the lines and areas with. I then move to my next larger size and so on until all of the areas are carved out. I then go back and cut out the tiniest smallest areas using the exacto blade. After I have finished the carving I flip the block over tap it gently to remove the shavings and then brush the block off with a paintbrush. I am now ready to print.

For **printing** I first cut my paper to one inch larger on each side than the block -- a 7x10 block would require a 8x11 sheet of paper. Squeeze out the ink onto a smooth surface -- glass or plexi -- and roll out a small amount smooth on the glass. Charge the brayer with ink. Now roll the ink onto the block -- first roll

vertically then horizontally -- this smoothes the
ink and insures that you roll the ink over the
entire block. Now print.

To print lay the paper on top of the inked block.
Gently press it down. Starting from one edge of
the paper rub in slow gentle but firm circles
until you have covered the entire block. Peel up
a corner and check to see that the image has
transferred completely. If the image hasn't rub
again in the places that haven't printed. I find
that it takes several inkings to get the first
good print.

If you don't have a brayer you can use a sponge
brush to ink the block. If you use a sponge brush
you can use a heavy acrylic paint to ink your
block.

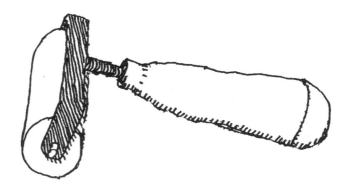

HOW TO:
Make your own paint brushes:

NEEDS:
· your hair   · embroidery thread   · strong glue
   · electrical tape   · wooded dowels

— make bundles of hair The longer the
better (you can always cut shorter but
can't add length.) It's also easier to
have the hair in each bundle to curl
the same way. [leave some at end] Now wrap
one end of bundle with thread as tightly
as possible. Put a small dot of
glue over the thread and smush together.

— Take dowel and stick it slightly into
the bottom of hair bundle. If using very
small dowels (such as BBQ skewers)
you may want to add another for support.

use a generous portion of glue on
joint.

— Wrap wet joint with thread and
roll in between your fingers making
sure to get the thread saturated with
the glue.

— Let dry)

— wrap the paintbrush with electrical
tape starting at top. Be really tight
at the top. Hide all string.

— Now pull on the bristles to get out
any loose hairs. Be thourough.

— Cut to desired length. — Ta-da!

MAKE YOUR OWN ENVELOPES!!!

SOMETIMES I MAKE MY OWN ENVELOPES TO MAIL THINGS IN. IT'S A NICE WAY TO PERSONALIZE WHATEVER YOU'RE MAILING. ALSO, THERE'S SO MUCH SCRAP PAPER THAT ALWAYS GET'S THROWN OUT. WHY NOT PUT IT TO SOME GOOD USE? HERE'S WHAT I DO:

GET A PIECE OF PAPER AND FOLD OVER THE EDGES ABOUT 1/4" - 1/2". NOW FOLD IT UP ALMOST IN HALF. GLUE THE FOLDED EDGES TO EACH OTHER. LET IT DRY AND YOU'VE GOT YOURSELF AN ENVELOPE!

WRITE A LETTER TO A FRIEND YOU HAVEN'T SEEN IN A WHILE AND STICK IT IN THERE. THEN PUT SOME GLUE ON THE EXTRA LITTLE FLAP PART AND FOLD IT OVER. NOW IT'S READY TO MAIL!

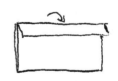

ANOTHER OPTION IF YOU CAN'T AFFORD 37¢ TO MAIL A LETTER BUT CAN AFFORD 23¢ TO MAIL A POSTCARD IS TO MAKE YOUR OWN POSTCARDS. JUST GET A SCRAP PIECE OF CARDSTOCK OR CARDBOARD (CEREAL BOXES WORK GOOD) AND CUT IT DOWN TO POSTCARD SIZE. NOW YOU'RE SET!

Make a Record Bowl

Did you know that not only are vinyl records fun to listen to, but you also turn them into bowls or flowerpots or ash trays! So, next time you're at the thrift store and you see all those crappy old records for sale for a quarter each, pick up a few and try this out.

In addition to a record, you'll need an oven, a baking pan, and a metal mixing bowl. Heat your oven to about 150 – 200 degrees. Place your mixing bowl upside down on your baking pan. Then put your record on top of the bowl. Place this in the oven. It should only take about 5 minutes for the record to get flexible. Be careful because it's hot! But also, you're going to need to work fast to shape your record into a bowl. You might want to wear some oven mitts or something. It hardens pretty fast, so if it gets too hard before you're done working it, just stick it back in the oven for a few minutes.

7 inches make good ash trays. 12 inches make good flowerpots.

To Make a Candle (or Torch)
Trina

Wax can easily catch on fire if not heated properly, so the best way to heat up wax is with a double boiler. You can buy double boiling pots for about $25, or you can just make your own. Bring some water to a boil in a regular pot, put your wax into a glass jar and set the jar into the hot water. Lower the heat and let the wax slowly melt within the jar. You may need to stir it occasionally. Using this double boiling method more evenly distributes the heat to the wax.

When your wax is ready, roll up a thin strip of cardboard – from a cereal box for example – and place it inside the rim of a metal lid such as a canning jar lid. Tape the outer flap of the cardboard down. Heat up some and drip it onto the cardboard. At first, just dribble a little bit of wax onto the cardboard then let it dry. Once dry fill it up the rest of the way with wax. This will help keep the wax from spilling out the edges. Once the wax dries you can light part of the cardboard and it will burn hot and bright for hours. You probably should place it in some sort of fireproof plate or bowl, because the wax will drip down the edges.

This "candle" creates a small bit of smoke and a flame that's about 6 – 8" tall, so it's recommended that you only burn it outdoors. It really functions more as a small torch than a candle, making for nice outdoor lighting. It might be worth experimenting with adding some citronella to the wax to create your own mosquito repellant torches. It also would probably work well to cook with on campouts.

① How to Hook A Rug by Corina Fastwolf

Rug hooking is simple + it's a great way to recycle old fabric. Here's what you need:

- A piece of burlap a bit bigger than the size of your finished piece

- 100% wool fabric. Go to churchsales, thrift stores, your closet etc. You want to have **long** strips of fabric so pants, skirts + blankets give you the most yardage for the buck. Wash the wool fabric on "HOT," then dry it in a hot drier. This will make the wool shrink a bit and make it seem a bit more, well, wooly.

- A rug hook (available at craft or yarn stores · get the plain kind, not the one with the latch) or a crochet Hook · I use a size 7 metal hook

- A big embroidery hoop helps stretch out the burlap and makes the project easier. I always see these at thrift stores so check there first before buying one at a craft store.

- A black magic marker, scissors, needle + thread

To get started draw the design of your rug on the burlap. Stick with simple outlines, blocking out which colors will go where in your head. Leave about 2" of burlap around the border for a "hem".

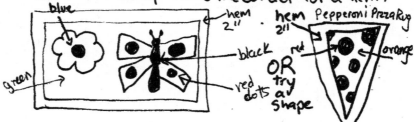

blue / green / hem 2" / hem 2" / Pepperoni Pizza Rug / black / red / orange / OR try a shape / red dots

② ★ Rug Hooking cont. ★

Now you need to tear the fabric into strips. The strips should be about ⅛–¼" wide. First you have to remove all hems, cuffs, collars etc. Break down the clothing so you have blocks of cloth with a straight edge.

For example:

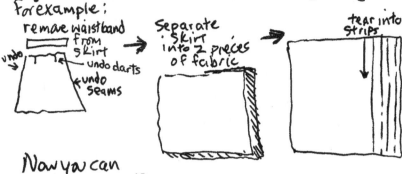

remove waistband from skirt
undo
undo darts
undo seams

Separate skirt into 2 pieces of fabric

tear into strips

Now you can start hooking. If you have an embroidery frame, frame up the section where you want to begin:

Stick your hook down thru the burlap, and pull up a loop of wool.

Then do it again in the next hole, and the next. You can hook in straight lines for an orderly appearance, or wherever you want for a more "swirled" effect. Keep going, until you use up the whole piece of wool. Pull the wool end up to the top side. Go back + pull the beginning wool end through to the top side too. This will keep the rug from unravelling. Then start with another wool strip - keep your loops a uniform height.

wool end / loops / wool end
burlap

TIPS

★ Hand dyed, patterned or plaid fabrics look cooler than all plain colors. Mix it up.

★ It's easier to do shapes first, + fill in background patterns later.

③ ✿ Rug Hooking Continued ✿

When you are finished hooking your rug, if you like you can cut off the tops of the loops to create a pile. Use scissors, and do it just like you were giving your rug a haircut. Or just leave the loops alone.

SNIP!

To finish your rug, turn it over to the backside. Trim the burlap to about 1", then make a hem, folding it in ½" and then another ½". Pin it with straight pins. Using heavy cotton thread, stitch it down. Burlap tends to unravel, so the double fold should help your rug stay together.

½" ½"

Hooked Rug

pinned hem

Backside of rug

You can also sew on a felt or burlap backing, or buy latex adhesive which you smear on the backside of your rug + which glues down your stitches.

For more ideas you can look at books on rug hooking in the library. Of course, you can use any kind of fabrics for your rugs, or mix and match. If you use cotton (like jeans) the loops of your rug will go flat (cotton doesn't have the same "bounce" as wool). One book I read suggested making a bath mat out of plastic bags. Just cut them into strips, hook 'em up + voila!!

Craft store will also provide you with ideas + materials but for best results I suggest recycling instead of buying.

If you want to start small try making a pillow cover, or a cat sleeping pad.
Good Luck! ♡ Corina
Fastwolf

PURRR

How To set up a Sewing Machine

a Sewing machine can be a real handy item - you can alter and repair thrift store finds, quickly peg pants, make your own clothes, quilts, bags, pillows, toys, hats and tons more.

Its fairly easy to get ahold of an old cheap second-hand singer: check out classifieds, flea markets or local bulletin boards. Plus, once you put the word out, you can never tell who se aunt may be getting rid of a machine. I got my 1960's singer from my boss's wife.

One tip would be to stay clear of the newer computer-chip run machines, stick with the simpler manual ones. Serious repairs are cheaper.

Here's really basic instructions for getting the machine set up and ready to go. The placement or look of certain parts may differ from brand to brand. But all machines tend to keep parts in generally the same area.

First off - how to get the bobbin all set-up.

To fill up a bobbin is simple
① make sure the needle is at its highest position (turn the hand wheel toward you)

② Either open up the throat-plate or the metal door on the side of the machine under the throat-plate. (some machines differ as to how to get to the bobbin case.)

③ Reach in and pull the latch on the bobbin case out to pull the whole thing out. The bobbin should just fall out of the bobbin case once you tip it.

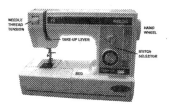

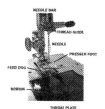

④ While winding the bobbin you need to stop the motion of the needle. (although i have skipped this part and everything turned out okay a few times)
Hold the hand wheel and turn the smaller wheel towards you. It will seem like you just loosened something. Now when you push on the foot pedal - the needle just stays in one place.

⑤ Put the empty bobbin on the spindle and move the bobbin winder lever to the right (it moves the spindle to the right also.)

⑥ Put a spool of thread on the spool pin. Wrap the thread around the bobbin winder tension bracket and wrap it around the middle of the empty bobbin.

⑦ Start the machine up with the floor pedal and if everything's right it should start filling up the bobbin with thread from the spool. If not re-check everything.

⑧ When the bobbin's full, cut the thread, move the bobbin winder lever back, take the bobbin off the spindle and re-tighten the smaller wheel on the hand wheel.

To put the bobbin back in the bobbin case follow these steps. It's easier to show these steps in pictures than words.

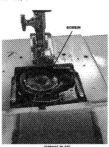
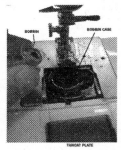

Don't worry, we're half there. Now it's time to THREAD THE MACHINE.

① Raise the needle to the highest position again.

② Put the spool of thread on the spool pin (if you just filled a bobbin it should already be in place)

③ Then lead the end of the thread thru the thread guide, needle thread tension regulator, take-up lever, down to the needle, thru the thread guides, and thru the eye of the needle. Always go from left to right thru the eye.

④ To gather up the bobbin thread, turn the hand wheel slowly towards yourself, while holding on to the end of the thread, keep turning until the needle passes in and back out of the throatplate. When it comes back out, it should have the bobbin thread hooped in with top thread. Pull on the top thread to lift it entirely out of the throatplate. Take both threads and pull till about 3" are from the pressure foot. Lay them to the right side. And the machine is finally set to go.

Straight stitch and zig zag are the two you'll use the most. On some machines you just set the stitch selector lever on whichever one you want and start sewing. But if your machine has things like needle position selector, stitch width, as well as stitch length selectors use the chart below to set them.

	NEEDLE POSITION	STITCH WIDTH	STITCH LENGTH
STRAIGHT STITCH	C (CENTER)	| FAR RIGHT	IF THE MATERIAL YOU'RE SEWING IS LIGHT-TO-MEDIUM HEAVINESS USE 12 TO 15 DENIM USE 10 TO 12
ZIG ZAG STITCH	C (CENTER) L OR R COME IN HANDY FOR BUTTONHOLES	⧠ FAR LEFT	FROM 6 TO THE FINE AREA FOR A TIGHT ZIGZAG PUT IT IN THE FINE AREA

REMEMBER TO LET YOUR IMAGINATION GO WILD AND MOST OF YOUR LEARNING WILL COME FROM TRIAL AND ERROR.

For further info on machine problem solving or sewing tips the library always has tons of books on the subject. Also, garage sales and thrift stores are good for scoring cheap books.

CORDially YOURS: A BRIEF INTRODUCTION TO CORD MAKING

Cord is used for tying, towing, rigging, netting, lashing, suspending, anchoring, and weaving (thread being slender cord). Because it is made cheaply by machines, it is often taken for granted. But not when it must be made by hand. A large bundle was worth a horse in trade to early Indians.

For millenia our ancestors made cord. I have taught hundreds of people how. All those about 4 years and older have learned within a few minutes.

Material for making into cord abounds. One estimate says 1,000 plants in North America furnish usable fibers. These include cattail, sedge, and rush leaf fibers (iris and grass leaves are shorter, thus require more splicing); flax, hemp, and stinging nettle stem fibers (after separating from the pith); some trees' inner bark fibers; and cotton's seed fibers. There are also animal fibers, such as wool. Additionally, discards such as paper bags and rags, can be made into cord.

Good candidates for testing are plants or materials you notice that resist tearing. Recently I tested sword-fern stems. Tho the fibers tended to break as I separated them from the pith, many were still several inches long, and made into strong cord.

I cut cattail close to the ground, and leave it lying in a dry place to dry.* If slow drying, I remove the leaves from the stems to increase air circulation. If I plan to later fit the leaves into plastic bags, I coil them when partly dry but still bendable without cracking. Then I let them dry further -- but not so dry that they are too brittle to handle. The leaves, or what you make from them, will keep indefinitely in the same kind of place where books remain free of mildew.

To soften, I soak cattail or sedge in plain water a minute or two; rushes about 5 min. (Room-temp water is fine, tho warmer water might speed softening.) Then I keep the leaves in a closed container, or wet towel, in a cool place (to retard spoiling) while moisture distributes evenly. About 12 hours may be best, but three hours or even less may suffice.

If using rags, I suggest beginners cut strips about a half inch wide; if paper; 3/4 inch wide and double over for tear resistance.

MAKING 2-PLY CORD -- WITHOUT a spindle

Hang your material on a projection. I'll refer to the material on one side as a "strand" even if it is numerous fibers, or more than one strip. (You may use more than one strip to get a fatter cord. Treat them all as if one.) Hold the strands as illustrated. The left strand is between the palm, and the little and ring fingers of the left hand. The right strand is between the thumb, and the pointer and middle fingers of the left hand.

Twist the right strand with the thumb and pointer finger of the right hand. The right thumb moves to the right. While the right hand twists, the left hand relaxes its grip on the right strand (only) to allow the twist to move up the material. (The left hand continues to hold the left strand.) Then the left hand clamps the right strand while the right hand returns to its starting position. (These directions will be easier to understand if you do it while you read them -- or better yet, while someone else reads them aloud.

Make 3 or 4 twists. Then pass the right strand to the left, OVER (or in front of) the left strand. The left strand moves to the right and becomes the right strand. That's it, just two steps: 1) twist to the right, and 2) pass over to the left. Repeat these 2 steps until your cord is as long as you want, or you start to run out of material and thus need to make a splice.

The dark strand is new material being spliced in.

TO IMPART TWIST, RIGHT THUMB MOVES RIGHT

PASS OVER TO THE LEFT (ANTI-CLOCKWISE)

TWIST IS CLOCKWISE

SPLICING. If you did not start with strands of unequal length, cut one strand now so it's several inches shorter than the other. This will avoid two splices opposite each other, which would result in a big lump.

Make your splice when the strand that's running out is on the left (see illustration). Start your splice when there are still a few inches of the old strand remaining, so that old and new overlap enough to securely hold in the new. Lay the new material over the old (as in the illustration) with a few inches sticking up, to be trimmed off after plying is finished.

Twist the right strand as usual, then pass it over both old and new material, treating them as one. The left strand (with the splice) has become the right strand. Twist old and new as one, and pass over as usual.

If your strands include more than one element (SEVERAL leaves, or strips, for added thickness, as opposed to only one; or numerous fibers), for a better splice do not splice in all elements at once. Instead, stagger the elements in the old strand (if not staggered, cut to make them so) and splice in only one or a few elements at a time.

MAKING CORD HEAVIER. To strengthen and thicken your cord, you may ply it again. First get it a bit over twice the length you want your finished cord to be. (Twist takes up some length.) Then wind from each end, to within a few feet of the middle, making two balls. A rubber band around each prevents unwinding. Hang the cord on a nail, one ball hanging down on either side. (The advantage of balls (versus loose cord on the floor): the balls rotate as you twist, thus resistance to twist does not build up. Nor is there tangling, because the balls move with you when strands exchange.)

Ply opposite to the first ply: right thumb moves LEFTward, and right strand passes UNDER left strand. Unwind from the balls as needed.

For rope stouter yet, ply again. (Instead of trying to remember the direction to twist, simply twist the cord. If it tightens, continue. If it loosens, twist the other way. Then, if you're twisting to the RIGHT, pass OVER to the left. If twisting to the LEFT, pass UNDER.

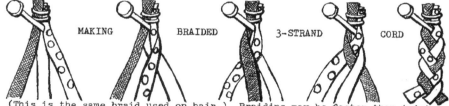

MAKING   BRAIDED   3-STRAND   CORD

(This is the same braid used on hair.) Braiding may be faster than twisting, and easier if material stiff. Twisted cord may be rounder and, if fibers short, stronger. The right strand is crossed over the middle strand. Then the left strand is crossed over the (newly become) middle strand. Repeat these two steps until done. (Whether you FOLD or BEND when crossing over, depends on stretchiness and what looks best. Begin any splice when the strand that's ending is in the middle. Lay the new material over it and proceed as usual, treating old and new as one. For tangle-free braiding, suspend the strands high enough so the ends are off the floor. If too long for that, wind into balls, each secured with a rubber band.

MAKING ROPE FROM BAILING TWINE. Farmers discard much (1-ply) twine, removed when hay is fed. Ply it repeatedly (as above) to get rope as thick as you want. A spindle will speed things up -- see "Twist Rags to Riches".

* Cord may be made immediately after harvesting the plants, but will have a loose twist after drying. To avoid this, plants are first dried, then prior to use, soaked only long enough to make pliable, which adds little water.

HOW TO MAKE A TAPE WALLET.

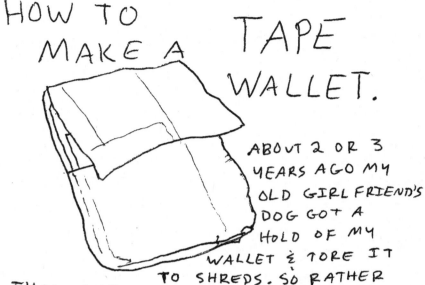

ABOUT 2 OR 3 YEARS AGO MY OLD GIRLFRIEND'S DOG GOT A HOLD OF MY WALLET & TORE IT TO SHREDS. SO RATHER THAN GOING OUT & BUYING A NEW WALLET I DECIDED I'D TRY TO MAKE MY OWN. I GOT A ROLL OF PACKING TAPE & WENT TO WORK. IT WAS REALLY EASY & HAS BEEN VERY DURABLE. IN FACT, I STILL USE THE SAME WALLET TO THIS VERY DAY. YOU CAN GO ABOUT MAKING YOURS HOWEVER YOU WANT, BUT HERE'S HOW I MADE MINE:

GET SOME TAPE. I USED CLEAR PACKING TAPE THAT'S ABOUT 2 INCHES WIDE, BUT A FRIEND OF MINE USED DUCT TAPE & THAT WORKED GREAT TOO.

FIRST OFF, I'D RECOMMEND MAKING THE 2 OUTER WALLS OF THE WALLET THAT MAKE THE POCKET TO HOLD $$$ BILLS IN. YOU CAN MAKE THIS BY GETTING 2 PIECES OF TAPE & STICKING THEM TO EACH OTHER (STICKY SIDES FACING EACH OTHER). JUST BUILD UP THE TAPE ON TOP OF ITSELF UNTIL IT'S SLIGHTLY LARGER THAN A DOLLAR BILL, & BE SURE THAT NONE OF THE STICKY SIDE IS EXPOSED.

NEXT YOU'LL WANT TO TAPE THESE 2 WALLS TOGETHER TO FORM THE $$$ POCKET. BE SURE TO TAPE IT REAL GOOD ON THE INSIDE & THE OUTSIDE LEAVING NO HOLES & NO EXPOSED STICKINESS.

NOW MAKE ANOTHER LITTLE TAPE WALL TO SERVE AS A POCKET TO KEEP YOUR LICENSE & LIBRARY CARD & WHATEVER ELSE YOU'VE GOT. TAPE THAT SUCKER ON THERE JUST LIKE YOU DID WITH THE OTHER PIECES.

NOW FOLD IT OVER AND THERE YOU HAVE IT. STICK IT SNUG IN YOUR BACK POCKET & BE THE ENVY OF ALL YOUR FRIENDS.

the d.iy-ification of

1. Style, because it is not a skill but an aesthetic, is inherently DIY:
everyone has it.
2. The Fashion Industry spends millions of dollars to have you believe
that it isn't; to sell your style back to you in small, ready-to-wear
packages; to design your desire.
3. Although ready-to-wear was at first called "the democratization of
style, as it made possible the buying of clothes by the
lower classes, mass production to-day has gotten out
of hand The fashion industry seems to be devouring
itself with such insid-ious practices
as sweatshop
labor,media control
and brand-name
hype.
4. By empowering
people to create their
own clothes, I hope to
aide in the self-destruct
ion of the industry and
make style more acces-
sible, important
and individual to
everyone.
5. So, I suggest you
arm yourself with a
sewing machine, some
thread and a good
pair of scissors.

style

Fabrics can be found
in many ways. From the
rearrangement of old clot
hes, or that of friends.
From thrift stores in the
form of sheets or other
linens. From textile du-
mpsters, tho only in big
cities and mostly in sm-
all scraps. From recycle
and reuse centers,etc...
   The sewing machine is
frustrating as all get-
out, at first. Some thin-
gs to watch for: don't
force the fabric thru. keep the tension near the
middle. don't rotate the
needle backwards. knitted
fabrics require a ball-
point needle. make sure to
put the presser foot down,
and threaded correctly. It
gets easier the more you
do it, really.
   The hardest part is
often cutting the fabric how
without a pattern but only
can take your fabric and pin
and mark it with chalk for
of clothing that you know
apart to see how they were
you want to be doing every

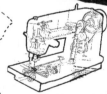

you want it, working
your awesome idea. Yo'
it directly on yoursel'
Or you can use a piece
a pattern. Take thing
Design based on what
where to cu
fits,as
made.
in sewing
ke pleats.
bigger one
things like
fabric toge
are useful,
day.

   Irons can be very helpful
before sewing them, or to ma-
but not a board or require a
over several newspapers. Other
ing (used to temporarily stick
stiffer), and fabric glue
necessary.
used to press seams
If you have an iron
you can put a towel
seamrippers,interfa
;ther, or to make it
but definitely not

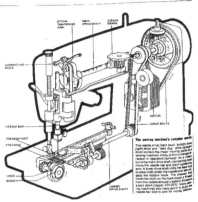

SEAMS - MACHINE

You can finish your seams any way the hell you want, but here are some common, sturdy ways of doing it:

1. Put the front, or'right' sides of the fabric together, and sew along the edge with a zigzag stitch.

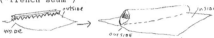

2. Put 'the backs together and sew along the edge, then reverse the fabric and sew a straight stitch to hide the seam. ("french seam")

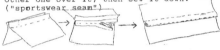

3. Put back or 'wrong' sides of fabric together and do a straight stitch. Cut one of the seam allowances and fold the other one over it, then sew it down. ("sportswear seam")

- (My) SEAMS -

BACKSTITCH

HEM OR SLIP STITCH

KNOT OR BLANKET STITCH

RUNNING STITCH

to KNOT THREADED NEEDLE, WRAP END OF THREAD IN LOOPS AROUND NEEDLE AND PULL IT DOWN

(even if you have claws, not hands)

TO KNOT OFF AT THE END OF A STITCH, MAKE A NORMAL STITCH AND THEN GO THRU IT TWICE.

Your local library will probably have books on sewing, or atleast books with machine trouble-shooting info like the one this diagram is from, "How things work in your home." For inspiration, I recommend books on quilts, traditional textile making such as strip weaving in Africa, and costume design. For info on the fashion industry I recommened No Sweat: Fashion, Free trade and the rights of garment workers, by Andrew Ross. "Fashion is Spinach" by Elizabeth Hawes and books by Angela McRobbie.

Mostly I recommend appreciating whatever teacher you can get in the subject, even if it is Mom. Through-out (western) history, sewing has been considered of little value- a "craft" when done by mothers and seamstresses, but an "art form" of high value when done by men as designers and tailors. It's time, I think, to open eyes with a broader definition of style.

Contact:

Live for Free,
po8148, Ann Arbor
MI, 48107

Fitted A-Line Skirt

①Measure Yourself

with a string and a ruler, or a measuring tape
if you have one. Be generous, you want it to
be comfortable.

A. your waist

B. your hips

C. the distance
between them

D. skirt length

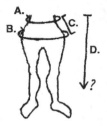

Supplies:

* measuring tape
(or string & a yardstick)

* **big paper** for a pattern... newspaper,
wrapping paper, whatever you have.

* **fabric.** You will know how much you
need after you make the pattern. You
can sometimes find fabric in second
hand stores- try to find a warehouse for
better selection & price.

* **zipper**   * sharp **scissors**.

* a razor blade or seam ripper would
also be nice.

② Make A Pattern

Use your measurements to draw this
shape on the big paper. Cut it out and put
it up to you to see if it seems right.

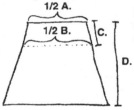

1/2 A.

1/2 B.   C.

D.

③ Getting the Fabric

Fabric generally comes in **45"** or **60"** width. Measure the bottom
of your skirt pattern. You will need twice this for the length plus
about 12 inches. The pattern will fit like this on the fabric:

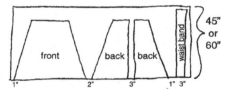

front   back   back

waist band

45"
or
60"

1"   2"   3"   1" 3"

④ Cutting the Skirt

①. Pin the pattern to the fabric, placing the bottom of the skirt on the edge of the fabric (this
will be your hem). Cut 1" larger than your pattern all the way around, so there will be room for
stitches. ②. Fold the pattern in half and cut out two of this shape. Leave 1" all the way around
each time. ③. Cut a long strip the length of your waist plus 2", and about 3" wide.

⑤ Putting it Together

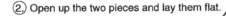

①. Pin the two back pieces together, right sides touching. Sew the middle
edge together one inch from the edge.

back

②. Open up the two pieces and lay them flat.

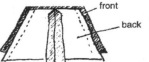

front

back

③. Pin this side to the front, right sides facing. Sew
them together leaving 1/2" edges. Start on the **bottom**
so your hem is **even**.

Fitted A-Line Skirt

continued...

⑥ Attaching the Waist Band

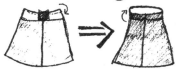

①. Fold that 3 inch strip in half the long way. Sew it together at the ends, making a loop. Make sure this is the same as the waist of the skirt.②. Turn the skirt body right side out. Pin the waistband on upside down with all the raw edges matching. Make sure the back seams line up. Sew all the way around 1/2" from the top.

⑦ Putting in the Zipper

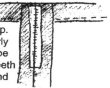

①. Turn the skirt inside out and lay it flat with the back seam facing up. ②. Pin the zipper **face down** on the middle of the seam.③. To properly sew in the zipper, it helps to have a zipper foot, or a foot that can be moved to the left or the right on your machine. Sew as close to the teeth of the zipper as you can down one side, a few times on the bottom, and then up the other side.

⑧ Liberating the Zipper

①. Turn the skirt right side out and lay it down with the back seam up.②. With a razor blade or seam ripper **CAREFULLY** take out the stitches above the zipper. **Stop** at the bottom of the zipper.

⑨ Making it work

Try it on. It fits? CONGRATULATIONS! **Too big?** Put it on inside out and pin where it needs to be fixed. Either resew the side seams or add darts. Cut away extra fabric only after you are certain it fits.**Too Small?** See if you can undo the side seams and sew closer to the edge.

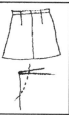

DARTS These are often in the back of skirts and dresses to allow for easier movement. They are V-Shaped to make the waist more narrow.

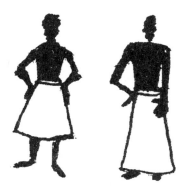

Also: Another way to make new clothes that fit is to use something you have as a template for a new pattern. Trace the pieces and make another.

How TO:
make a bikini out of bandanas:
NEEDS:
- 5 Bandanas
- needle & thread or saftey pins

TOP

- tie two ends together
- now fold each in half.
- roll up 3rd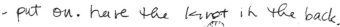
- tie each end of the 3rd
to the folded

- put on. have the knot in the back.
- now tie in front!

BOTTOMS

- Fold the last two into triangles
- Tie at two corners
- stick one leg through the hole
created
- then tie remaining corners
in knot.

* You may want to secure joints
by sewing them or pinining w/
Saftey pins.

* You may not want a knot in crotch
area. In such case you must sew that
joint together FLAT.

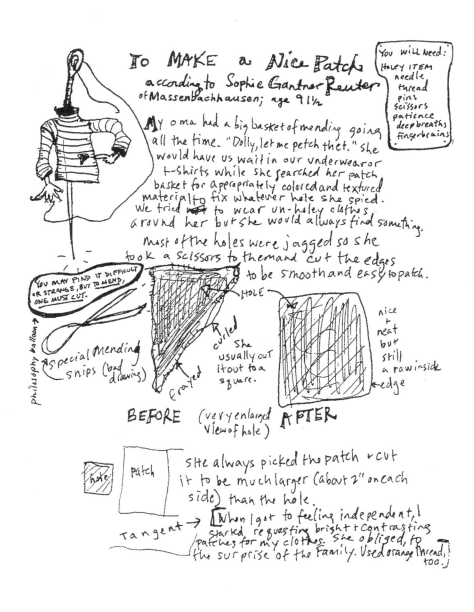

To MAKE a Nice Patch
according to Sophie Gantner Reuter
of Massenbachhausen; age 91½

YOU WILL NEED:
HOLEY ITEM
needle
thread
pins
scissors
patience
deep breaths
fingerbrains

My oma had a big basket of mending going
all the time. "Dolly, let me petch thet." She
would have us wait in our underwear or
t-shirts while she searched her patch
basket for a peropriately colored and textured
material to fix whatever hole she spied.
We tried not to wear un-holey clothes
around her but she would always find something.

Most of the holes were jagged so she
took a scissors to them and cut the edges
to be smooth and easy to patch.

YOU MAY FIND IT DIFFICULT
OR STRANGE, BUT TO MEND,
ONE MUST CUT.

Philosophy balloon →

A special mending
snips (bad drawing)

HOLE

curled

frayed

She
usually cut
it out to a
square.

nice
+
neat
but
still
a raw inside
edge

BEFORE (very enlarged
view of hole)   AFTER

hole   patch

She always picked the patch + cut
it to be much larger (about 2" on each
side) than the hole.

Tangent →   When I got to feeling independent, I
started requesting bright + contrasting
patches for my clothes. She obliged, to
the surprise of the family. Used orange thread,
too.

Then she would loosely pin the patch behind the hole on the "wrong" (inside-outside) of the shirt or pants she was mending.

Next (this was the hard part) she would roll the raw edges of the hole in order to make a tiny hem and deftly pin it down. This is tricky. Be patient, you can do it. I roll the edge in with my 1st finger and thumb, then hold the hem in place with my thumb while I slip in a pin. She used lots of pins. Pinned the whole thing down. This part all happens on the "right" (rightside out) side of the shirt pants whatever.

please be patient

OK. So now it's time to sew. The thread, I like to keep it sort of short because I find it catches on all the pins. My oma sewed the inside part of the patch with a tight over hand stitch. Most of the time I could barely see the stitches. Then she basted the edges of the patch to the short pants whatever. She was fast. "Dere you go, Dolly," she would say after 15 minutes. It takes me about an hour. I'd have to say pinning it a before hand is the key. Safety pins work OK as pins if yer short. Try it a lot. Its satisfying. Don't use rotten patch material, no matter how pretty. And my name ain't Dolly, it's Mo

wrong

opinion

A GOOD TIME TO PATCH: RAIN WEATHER GOOD COMPANY

"right" side

patch material

pins

raw edge

rolled hem

basting stitch "RIGHT" SIDE

patch edge as imagined through material.

Unstink your Socks

I USUALLY WEAR MY SOCKS 2 OR 3 DAYS IN A ROW. AFTER A WHILE THEY GET A LITTLE CRUSTY ON THE BOTTOM & START TO STINK PRETTY BAD. I HEARD THAT THE BACTERIA THAT CAUSES THE STINK WILL DIE WHEN EX-POSED TO UV RAYS SO I TOOK A FEW OF MY NASTY OLD SOCKS & LAID THEM IN THE SUN FOR A COUPLE DAYS. THEY ALSO GOT SPRINKLED ON A BIT TOO & WHEN I WENT TO RETRIEVE THEM THEY DIDN'T STINK ANYMORE! OF COURSE THE BOTTOMS WERE STILL CRUSTY, BUT, HEY, YOU CAN'T BE TOO PICKY.

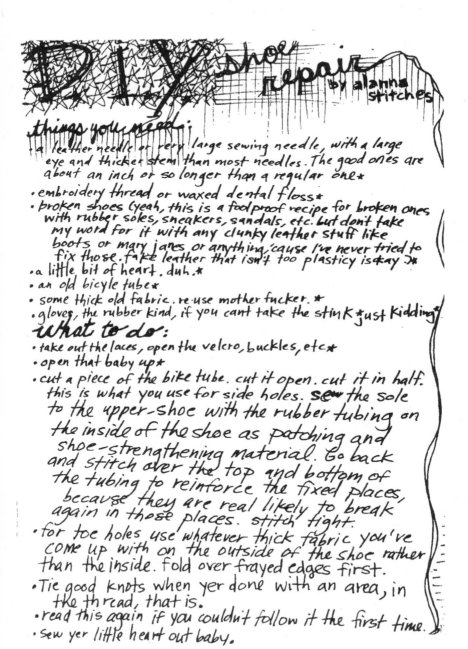

D.I.Y. shoe repair
by alanna stitches

things you need:

- a leather needle or very large sewing needle, with a large eye and thicker stem than most needles. The good ones are about an inch or so longer than a regular one*
- embroidery thread or waxed dental floss*
- broken shoes (yeah, this is a foolproof recipe for broken ones with rubber soles, sneakers, sandals, etc. but don't take my word for it with any clunky leather stuff like boots or mary janes or anything, 'cause I've never tried to fix those. fake leather that isn't too plasticy is okay)*
- a little bit of heart. duh.*
- an old bicyle tube*
- some thick old fabric. re-use mother fucker. *
- gloves, the rubber kind, if you cant take the stink *just kidding*

what to do:
- take out the laces, open the velcro, buckles, etc*
- open that baby up*
- cut a piece of the bike tube. cut it open. cut it in half. this is what you use for side holes. sew the sole to the upper-shoe with the rubber tubing on the inside of the shoe as patching and shoe-strengthening material. Go back and stitch over the top and bottom of the tubing to reinforce the fixed places, because they are real likely to break again in those places. stitch tight.
- for toe holes use whatever thick fabric you've come up with on the outside of the shoe rather than the inside. fold over frayed edges first.
- Tie good knots when yer done with an area, in the thread, that is.
- read this again if you couldn't follow it the first time.
- sew yer little heart out baby.

How to Make Stencils
Matte Resist

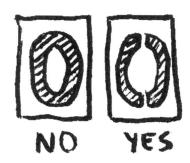

NO   YES

1. Come up with a design, but remember that you can't have "islands" such as the middle of an "O" or "R." You can use straight lines to connect the islands, or you can disguise it a little by making what appear to be slight flaws.

2. Transfer your design to a piece of cardboard or a transparency. One free resource for stencil cardboard is Priority Mail envelopes or similar cardboard envelopes that can be found at FedEx mailing stations. You can draw your design straight onto the cardboard or transparency. Also, thinner cardboard can be cut down to 8.5" x 11" and run through a photocopier. Try to keep the design toward the middle of the cardboard.

3. Using an incredibly sharp x-acto knife or other blade cut out the design. A dull knife will end up ripping the cardboard and cause a lot of problems.

4. Spray-paint works best with cardboard stencils. Just place the stencil over whatever you want it on and spray a coat of paint. You can't use spray-paint with transparency stencils because the chemicals in the paint will melt the plastic. I've found that acrylic paints work well with transparencies. Just dab it through the stencil using a sponge or brush. It takes very little paint to make it look nice. Too much will make the design run and look real blobby.

5. To preserve your stencil, dab any excess paint off before it dries. With transparency stencils you can also rinse excess paint off with water.

6. It has been suggested to me that when stenciling on patches and shirts you should iron the paint for a few minutes to heat-set it so it doesn't fade.

Stencil Folder
Luka Rubinioni

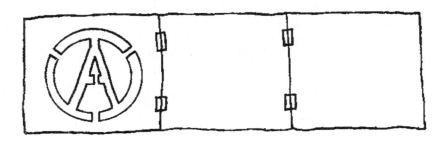

    You can make an advanced version of a cardboard stencil that won't dribble or get on your clothes when you transport it. You'll need two sheets of cardboard about the same size as your stencil. Tape these two pieces together, then tape one edge of one of these pieces to your stencil. You can hide your stencil inside this "folder" and open it easily whenever you want to use it. This device will not only help you safely transport your stencil, but will also conceal it in a nondescript form. This is very important in some places such as Yugoslavia where you can get 1 month in jail for doing political graffiti. Another way to remain unnoticed when doing graffiti is to wear a long sleeve shirt and hold the can of spray-paint up your sleeve.

Simple Puppets

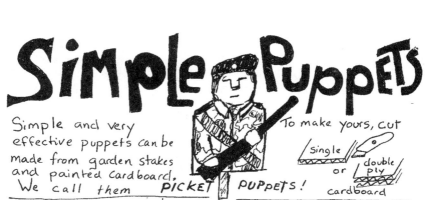

Simple and very effective puppets can be made from garden stakes and painted cardboard. We call them **PICKET PUPPETS!**

To make yours, cut

single

or double ply

cardboard

into the desired shape.

Simple is best

Tack garden stake to cardboard

secure flimsy bits with lathe (1/4 x 1 1/2")

Sand or tape handle smooth 1'x2'

paint

or even add fabric like camouflage or guatemalan weaving

for a fancier version: cut 2 cardboard images

tack to stick

and staple edges closed

then paint either

front & back

OR

the same

2 or 3 people can make large numbers of these puppets very quickly in an assembly line fashion.

CUT   STAPLE   PAINT

Picket puppets are most powerful when a large group of them appears together. Either all alike:

1000 crosses, 200 ears of corn.

or variations on a theme:

the 42 martyrs of Acteal

Simple but co-ordinated "drill team" movements look great

Special effects are limited only by your imagination Try swinging arms - googly eyes - chattering teeth sound effects..

for November the designs we suggest are: soldiers, religious, students, skulls, indigenous people, corn and anything else you can dream up.

GIANT PUPPETS

Our first puppet was the 12' Virgin of Guadalupe - you may have seen her at previous SOAW events. We think she's great and want to share how we made her. Obviously your puppet will have its own quirks and innovations.

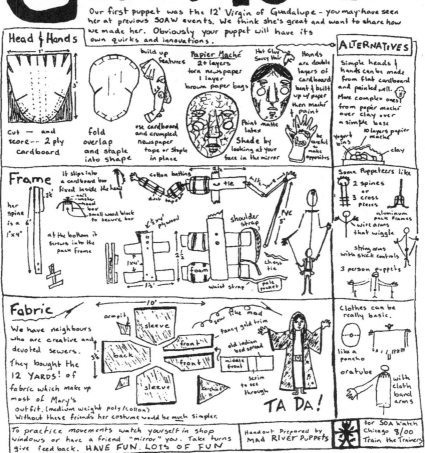

Head & Hands

Cut — and score-- 2 ply cardboard

fold overlap and staple into shape

build up features

use cardboard and crumpled newspaper tape or staple in place

Papier Maché
2+ layers torn newspaper
1 layer brown paper bags

Hot Glue Saucy Hair

Paint matte latex

Shade by looking at your face in the mirror

Hands are double layers of cardboard bent & built up w/ paper then maché paint

be careful to make opposites

ALTERNATIVES

Simple heads & hands can be made from flat cardboard and painted well. More complex ones from papier maché over clay over a simple base

Yogurt tins

10 layers papier maché

clay

Frame

her spine is a 6' 1"x4"

it slips into a cardboard box fixed inside the head

nail washer wood boot small wood block to secure box

at the bottom it screws into the pack Frame

cotton batting

tie

dust tape

shoulder strap

plywood ½"x¾"

1"x¾"

foam

chest tie

waist strap

pole pocket

Some Puppeteers like

2 spines or 3 cross pieces

aluminum pack frames wire arms that wiggle

string arms with stick controls

3 person puppets

Fabric

We have neighbours who are creative and devoted sewers.

They bought the 12 YARDS! of fabric which make up most of Mary's outfit. (medium weight poly/cotton)

Without these friends her costume would be much simpler.

armpit

sleeve

back

front

front

middle front

sew like mad

fancy gold trim

old indian bed spread

scrim to see through

kerchief

sleeve

TA DA!

Clothes can be really basic.

like a poncho

oratube

with cloth band arms

To practice movements watch yourself in shop windows or have a friend "mirror" you. Take turns give feedback. HAVE FUN. LOTS OF FUN

Handout Prepared by MAD RIVER PUPPETS

for SOA Watch Chicago 8/00 Train the Trainers

FLAGS

To find your affinity group in a crowd of several thousand having an identifiable marker up above the crowd is a big help. Your flag can be as simple as a T-shirt, pillow case or coloured streamers on a pole. Or it can be as elaborate as you wish.

For the pole, bamboo is cheap, light, strong but easy on the hands. Garden stakes, brooms or whatever else you have are fine. Just get your image UP.

To support your pole a length of sheet about 5'x6" knotted and duct taped to a tin can works great

Your "flag" does not need a pole. Try a very tall hat or a bouquet of helium balloons. A giant puppet, a stilt-walker. Flags of any kind draw attention and confer instant authority! Every affinity group should have one.

TOOLS and TECHNIQUES

Cardboard
Double-ply is really stiff - good for flat things.

Cereal Boxes are flimsy but OK for detail work.

This kind is super flexible and fun but pretty rare. SINGLE-PLY IS THE GREATEST!

STRONG this way

bend it shape it staple it build a new friend

flexible this way

Fasteners
Heavy duty staple pliers (with a pointy bottom jaw) attach cardboard to cardboard. Staples fold to hold pieces together. Best of all they can attach a flat piece to a 3-D object.

Heavy duty tacker staplers stick cardboard to wood. Staples go in straight ∏

Papier Maché
Mix up some wallpaper paste or cook yummy wheat paste = flour + H_2O (mice love it) Dampen strips or squares of torn paper with paste, apply to surface. begin w/newspaper, finish w/brown paper. try to do 2 or 3 layers at a time. For big projects laminate 2 or 3 sheets of paper together, let it dry, then tear and apply.

Boxes of cardboard made to fit the frame and secured inside puppet head or hands make disassembly easy and prevent wobbling.

Washers can be made by cutting circles out of plastic containers and will keep nails from pulling through cardboard.

latex paint is easy to get free and dries fast. Use matte not gloss.

Duct tape is the greatest BUT expensive & easy to over use. Will a staple or masking tape work as well?

Some really basic self-explanatory stuff: white glue wood glue masking tape box knife, fabric scissors, paint, brushes, buckets, rags, markers, drill, saw, pliers, safety pins, foam, PVC, hammer, screwdriver, string, wire, sheets, inner tubes, needle, thread, glue gun, wood, plastic bags, screws, nails.

DO NOT BE DAUNTED! WE HAVE MADE A GREAT PUPPET FROM PAPER, CARDBOARD, TAPE, GLUE, PAINT, A KNIFE, A STICK AND A SHEET. YOU CAN TOO.

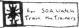

by MAD RiVER! PUPPETS   for SOA Watch Train the Trainers

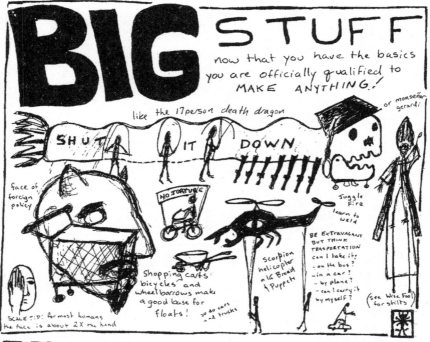

Where can I learn more?

Wise Fool Basics $10 – 15 (essential)
2633 Etna St. Berkeley, CA 94704
(415) 905 - 5958
www.zeitgeist.net/wfca/wisefool.htm

68 Ways to Make Really Big Puppets
by Puppeteers' Coop, available through $4
Bread and Puppets' Catalogue
753 Old, Heights Rd. Glover VT 05839

Drums and Demonstrations $4
Super Sonic Samba School (619) 281-1066
334, Gregory St. San Diego CA 92104
http:// ssss.console.net   Sonigueiro@aol.com

Puppet Cookbook $25 (worth every penny)
In the Heart of the Beast (612) 721-2535
1500 East Lake St. Minneapolis MN 55407

Games for Actors and Non-Actors
Augusto Boal, Routledge, 1992.

Engineers of the Imagination
Tony Coult & Baz Kershaw, Methuen, 1983.
out of print but a prize if you can find it

ACO Staple & Abrasive Co.
347 Aspen Ave. South San Francisco, CA 94050
PO Box 2456 SF, CA 94124 (415) 589-9920
is where Wise Fool orders Rapid·31 staplers

We at **Mad River**! have borrowed freely from all these sources for our handouts. THANKS ALL

How to Wheatpaste
Adapted from a flyer by the Lesbian Avengers.

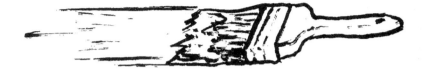

Wheatpasting flyers and posters is a great way to spread ideas beyond the inner circle of your subculture and close friends and, instead, get them out to the public. Posters and flyers that are wheatpasted to just about any surface will stay up until someone scrapes them off. Stapling posters isn't as permanent as wheatpasting and is becoming less and less of an option in many modern cities where wooden telephone poles have all been removed.

The first step, before you can start the actual wheatpasting, is to make a really great, eye-catching flyer. There are numerous styles of effective flyer design, but some basic things to keep in mind are: good clear images, large easy to read lettering, and a sense of humor. People tend to give more time and thought to flyers that make them laugh rather than condemning them.

To make your own paste, mix one cup of flour with 1 ½ cups of water. Stir the mixture well to remove any lumps. On a stove, heat this mixture to a boil until it thickens. You may need to add more water, and stir for a bit, until it turns into a thick, clear goop. Cook on low heat for about a half hour, regularly stirring it to avoid burning. The paste expands a bit when cooking, so you may need to experiment to get the best consistency. Some wheatpasters, instead of making their own, prefer to buy wallpaper paste from hardware stores because it is more consistent and is just as effective as homemade paste.

Now it's time to put your paste into action. Smear the paste onto the surface where you want your poster using a large, wide brush or putty knife. Also smear the paste onto the back of your poster, then stick it up. You may also want to apply the paste over the front of your poster too. This helps it stick and also gives it a protective coating so it will last longer. It's important to make sure you paste the corners of your poster sufficiently or else it will be easier for someone to tear it down.

Some people use an empty dishwashing soap bottle to carry their paste around and just squeeze it directly onto their brush. Others carry it around in a small bucket. Wheatpasting is best done with two people (one to handle paste, another to handle the posters).

how to make glue from pine sap:
first of all collect some sap from any
kind of pine tree (spruce and fir work too)
But the x glob of sapin an old tin can and melt
itover a fire. Let the sap boil for a few seconds
then add a pinch or two of ashes from the fire
The ashes make the sap harden up once it cools.
the more ashes you k add the harder (more brittle)
it will get. Once the ashes are mixed in you are
ready to use.it. Simply apply and allow to cool.

HAND DRILL FIRE:
HAND DRILL FIRE:
OK, this is one of the most basic ways of
making a fire by friction. You will need a
long straight stalk 2-3 ft. long that is
good and dry. Mullein stalks are great for
this, so are elderberry. You will also need a
baseboard which is what the stalk will be
drilling into to make a coal. This should
be made from a medium hard wood like cedar,
cottonwood, aspen, sassafrass, or birch.
Pines are terrible and so are hardwoods
like oak and hickory. Make an indentation
in the baseboard with a knife about the
width of the stalk so tha it won't pop out
of the notch. Now you will burn a hole into
the baseboard by twisting the stalk back and
forth between your hands until you have enough
of an indentation so that the stalk won't pop
out easily while twisting. Now you will cut
a notch into the hole about an xixk eighth of

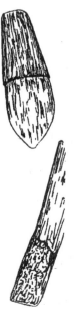

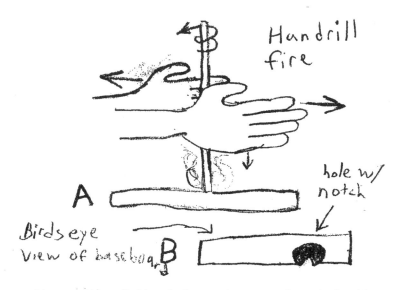

Handrill fire

A

hole w/ notch

Birdseye View of baseboard B

the width of the hole and goes almost to the
center but not quite as illustrated in fig.B2B
This notch is made to allow the wood dust to
pile up which will eventually become a coal
once it is heated up enough. Now you're ready
to rock. Start twisting the stalk by running
it between the entire length of your hands,
so that the stalk rabiply twists back and forth
drilling into the baseboard. It's really
important to use your whole hand so that you
get enough friction. While twisting make sure
to put lots of downward pressure too. Your hands
will get to the butx bottom of the stalk quickly.
hold the bottom of the stalk in place with one hand
while bringing the other up to the top and start

drilling away again. Eventually you get smoke
and if your lucky you will soon have a coal in

the wood dust that has accumulated in the notch.
Pick up the coal with the blade of your knife

and place in a nest of x dried grass or bark.
blow until the coal grows into a flame.

BOW DRILL FIRE:
This is the same idea as the hand drill
with a few extra components. In some
respects bow drill is easier but there's
more components so there are more ways you
can fuck up. The parts are: 1. Bow, a two foot
or so long stick, with a string tied to both ends.
2. Spindle, about the length xxx of your hand
made from woods recommended for baseboard in handrill
section. XXX Should be about 1/2 inch diameter
3. Baseboard, same as handrill. 4. Hand grip,
this is for holding the spindle down. Use
bone or smooth stone like quartz if possible.
Hardwoods will work well too. The idea is to
have as little friction as possible on this
part.
So make an indentation and notch like you
do in a hand drill fire. Now you will wrap
the cord of the bow once around the spindle
so that the string is very tight. Put the
top of the spindle in the hole in the handhold
and the bottom of the spindle in the baseboard
while pushing down with the handhold. Move
the bow back and forth so that it spins the
spindle while still applying lots of downward
pressure. Keep spinning until you get
smoke and coal.

bow drill in action

← smoke!

troubleshooting: I realize that this is easier
said then done. It takes a lot of practice
and patience. Here's a few hints though
1. If xxwood dust is not building up
in the notch you may need to make the notch
bigger
2. If the spindle keeps popping out of the
hole you may need to make a smaller notch
or the hole may be too close to the edge.
3. experiment with different combos of wood.
a spindle and baseboard made of the same type
of wood generally works well but there other
combos which may work better.

Rubbing Alcohol Campstove

This is a really simple stove that I like to carry along when I'm camping in case the woods too wet to start a fire. All you need is a tin can and some rubbing alcohol. Poke holes towards the top of the can all the way around for ventilation. Pour in alcohol to just below the holes. Light it! Prop your pot over it with rocks or something and your cookin'! Alcohol won't light well if it's cold. If thats the case put the container of alcohol down your trousers about a 1/2 hour before you need it. Your body heat will warm it up. You may want a funnel to pour xtra alcohol into container. Also something to block the wind.

Happy Camping

Poorly drawn flame that looks like X-mas tree →

Ventilation holes

Pork N Beans

Wild Food

Info for this article is based on my own personal experience, and also adapted from an article by Matt Wallace in his zine Tar and Feathers #1, and the wonderful book *Edible Plants of the Gulf South* by Andy Allen, Charles Allen, and Harry Winters. Illustrations by Andy Allen.

Cattail

Cattails are very plentiful all around the Gulf-South of the US. I don't know if they grow elsewhere, but I assume they do well in moist and warm areas, specifically in swampy areas. You can gather and eat them year round, and they provide a lot of edible food, and are supposed to be high in protein. In the early spring the young shoots will start to come

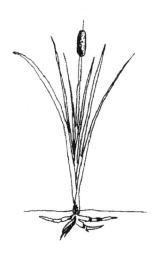

up. These can be gathered and eaten raw or cooked like asparagus. Some people actually call this "Cossack Asparagus." They're great in stir-fry too. Early in the summer the green flower stalk (the part that eventually turns into a white poofball later in the year) can be collected, cooked, and eaten as well. Eventually the flower heads get real tough and start making pollen. You can collect this pollen by sticking the head in a bag and shaking it. The pollen will fall off. You can then use this as a nutritious additive to mix into flour or as a topping sprinkled on any kind of food.

Dandelion

Dandelions are a common weed that can be found growing in almost any man-made open area – lawns, fields, parks, along roadsides, etc. The flowers typically bloom in the late winter or early spring. Every part of the dandelion is edible, and due to their prolific presence, they make for a great wild food source. The 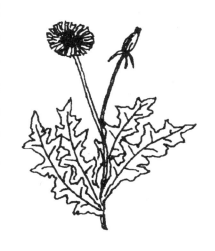 leaves can be used in salads. They're better when they're young and small. As the leaves age and grow they develop more bitterness, but are still edible. They can also be cooked as a green. Dandelion roots can also be eaten either raw or cooked, but again, they're better earlier, and they get tougher as they age. You can also roast the roots to make a caffeine-free coffee substitute. The flowers, too, can be eaten raw in salads, or cooked. The flowers can also be used to make a tea or even wine by simply steeping them in hot water for an hour or so to extract the flavor. Winemaking instructions can be found elsewhere.

Thistle

My in-laws have, for a long, long time, harvested and eaten thistle that grew out behind the back of their house. Thistle is best when it's harvested early. As it gets older, it gets tougher and harder to eat. They look very intimidating at first because

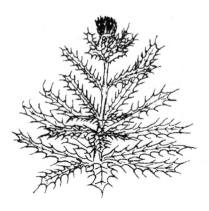

they're covered in big, pointy, scary looking leaves. All you have to do is bring a long knife with you when you're harvesting and slice off all the leaves before grabbing the plant. Once the leaves are gone you have a nice stalk that makes a good celery substitute that can be eaten raw or cooked as a veggie. The roots can also be pulled up, boiled, and eaten.

Sorrel

Sorrel leaves look similar to clover leaves. They're small, round, green, and have 3 leaves per stem. The difference is that sorrel is edible and very tangy! It makes a great addition to salads, adding a strong zest to the mix. If you pull up the root you can plant sorrel in a pot and grow it in your own home for regular use.

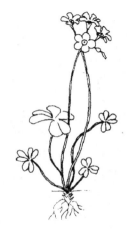

MY GARDEN

I JUST GOT STARTED ON MY OWN PERSONAL GARDEN. I'M GOING WITH THE SQUARE FOOT APPROACH AGAIN THIS YEAR. I DON'T REMEMBER IF I'VE WRITTEN ABOUT THIS BEFORE. THE IDEA IS TO MAXIMIZE THE USE OF SPACE. ROW GARDENS WERE DESIGNED TO MAKE PLANTING, WEEDING & CULTIVATING OF LARGE GARDENS EASIER. ROWS ARE MADE FOR GETTING CULTIVATORS AND OTHER MACHINES DOWN. IF YOU GROW A SMALL GARDEN YOU DON'T NEED ROWS. GROWING WITHOUT ROWS ALSO MAKES WEEDING EASIER, BECAUSE YOU DON'T HAVE A LOT OF OPEN SPACE, AND THE PLANTS SHADE OUT THE WEEDS. YOU ALSO USE LESS WATER, BECAUSE YOU WATER JUST THE PLANTS, NOT THE ROWS. PERSONALLY I THINK THEY LOOK BETTER TOO; THEY'RE FULL OF PLANTS WITH NO OPEN SPACES.

TO GET RID OF ROWS, YOU JUST NEED TO BE ABLE TO REACH ALL YOUR PLANTS, WITHOUT WALKING IN YOUR GARDEN. A 4 FOOT WIDTH ENSURES YOU CAN REACH THE MIDDLE FROM BOTH SIDES. IF YOU HAVE A LARGER GARDEN, YOU CAN USE PATHS. MY FIRST YEAR I PUT DOWN BOARDS TO WALK ON.

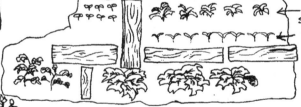

← I WAS STILL DOING ROWS THE YEAR I USED WOOD PATHS.

A BETTER WAY IS TO BUILD RAISED BEDS, WHICH IS WHAT I'VE DONE THE PAST TWO YEARS. YOU BUILD THE BEDS FOUR FEET WIDE, AND AS LONG AS YOU WANT. PATHS BETWEEN THEM SHOULD BE AT LEAST 2 FEET WIDE TO GIVE YOU ROOM TO WORK. LAST YEAR I BOUGHT 10" WIDE BOARDS, BECAUSE I WAS PUTTING THE BOXES ON TOP OF A GARDEN THAT HAD ALREADY BEEN TILLED. THIS YEAR I DIDN'T WANT TO TILL, AND I HAVE CLAY SOIL WHICH IS REALLY HARD TO GARDEN IN, SO I BOUGHT 12" WIDE BOARDS. THE BOXES ARE VERY EASY TO BUILD. 10"x2" & 12"x2" BOARDS COME IN 6, 8, 10 & 12 FOOT LENGTHS AT MOST LUMBER YARDS. MANY WILL CUT A FEW BOARDS FOR FREE, SO IF YOU WANT TO DO A 10'x4' BOX (WHICH IS WHAT I DID THIS YEAR) YOU JUST BUY TWO 10' LENGTHS, AND HAVE THEM CUT AN 8' FOOT LENGTH IN HALF FOR YOU. (OR YOU CAN CUT IT YOURSELF) THEN JUST NAIL OR SCREW IT ALL TOGETHER. I PREFER SCREWS BECAUSE THEY HOLD LONGER, BUT FOR CONVENIENCE' SAKE I USED NAILS THIS YEAR. I'LL PROBABLY ADD SCREWS LATER. I ALSO ADDED A SCRAP 2"x2" & 1"x6" IN THE MIDDLE TO KEEP IT FROM BOWING OUT UNDER THE WEIGHT OF THE SOIL.

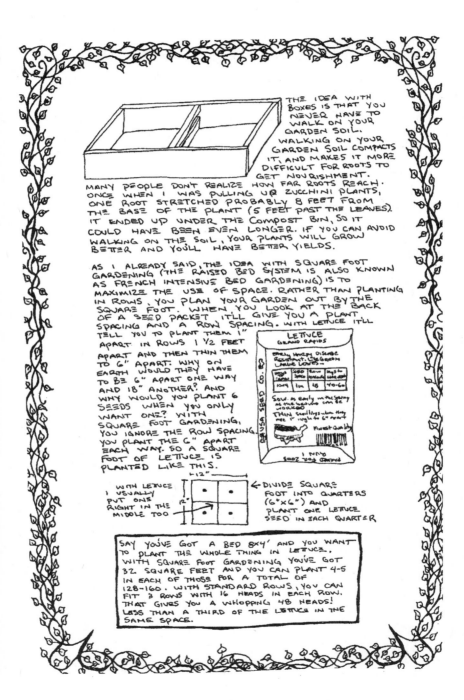

THE IDEA WITH BOXES IS THAT YOU NEVER HAVE TO WALK ON YOUR GARDEN SOIL. WALKING ON YOUR GARDEN SOIL COMPACTS IT, AND MAKES IT MORE DIFFICULT FOR ROOTS TO GET NOURISHMENT.

MANY PEOPLE DON'T REALIZE HOW FAR ROOTS REACH. ONCE WHEN I WAS PULLING UP ZUCCHINI PLANTS, ONE ROOT STRETCHED PROBABLY 8 FEET FROM THE BASE OF THE PLANT (5 FEET PAST THE LEAVES). IT ENDED UP UNDER THE COMPOST BIN, SO IT COULD HAVE BEEN EVEN LONGER. IF YOU CAN AVOID WALKING ON THE SOIL, YOUR PLANTS WILL GROW BETTER AND YOU'LL HAVE BETTER YIELDS.

AS I ALREADY SAID, THE IDEA WITH SQUARE FOOT GARDENING (THE RAISED BED SYSTEM IS ALSO KNOWN AS FRENCH INTENSIVE BED GARDENING) IS TO MAXIMIZE THE USE OF SPACE. RATHER THAN PLANTING IN ROWS, YOU PLAN YOUR GARDEN OUT BY THE SQUARE FOOT. WHEN YOU LOOK AT THE BACK OF A SEED PACKET IT'LL GIVE YOU A PLANT SPACING AND A ROW SPACING. WITH LETTUCE IT'LL TELL YOU TO PLANT THEM 1" APART IN ROWS 1 1/2 FEET APART AND THEN THIN THEM TO 6" APART. WHY ON EARTH WOULD THEY HAVE TO BE 6" APART ONE WAY AND 18" ANOTHER? AND WHY WOULD YOU PLANT 6 SEEDS WHEN YOU ONLY WANT ONE? WITH SQUARE FOOT GARDENING, YOU IGNORE THE ROW SPACING. YOU PLANT THE 6" APART EACH WAY. SO A SQUARE FOOT OF LETTUCE IS PLANTED LIKE THIS.

LETTUCE
GRAND RAPIDS

EARLY HARDY DISEASE RESISTANT. LITE GREEN LARGE LEAVES —

	SEED DEPTH	ROW SPACING	DAYS TO GERMINATION
1049	1 IN	18	40-60

SOW AS EARLY IN THE SPRING AS THE GROUND CAN BE WORKED

THIN SEEDLINGS WHEN THEY ARE 1" HIGH TO 6" APART

Finest Quality

PACKED FOR 2005
MFD 1

REUSA SEED CO.

WITH LETTUCE I USUALLY PUT ONE RIGHT IN THE MIDDLE TOO

← DIVIDE SQUARE FOOT INTO QUARTERS (6"x6") AND PLANT ONE LETTUCE SEED IN EACH QUARTER

SAY YOU'VE GOT A BED 8x4' AND YOU WANT TO PLANT THE WHOLE THING IN LETTUCE. WITH SQUARE FOOT GARDENING YOU'VE GOT 32 SQUARE FEET AND YOU CAN PLANT 4-5 IN EACH OF THOSE FOR A TOTAL OF 128-160. WITH STANDARD ROWS, YOU CAN FIT 3 ROWS WITH 16 HEADS IN EACH ROW. THAT GIVES YOU A WHOPPING 48 HEADS! LESS THAN A THIRD OF THE LETTUCE IN THE SAME SPACE.

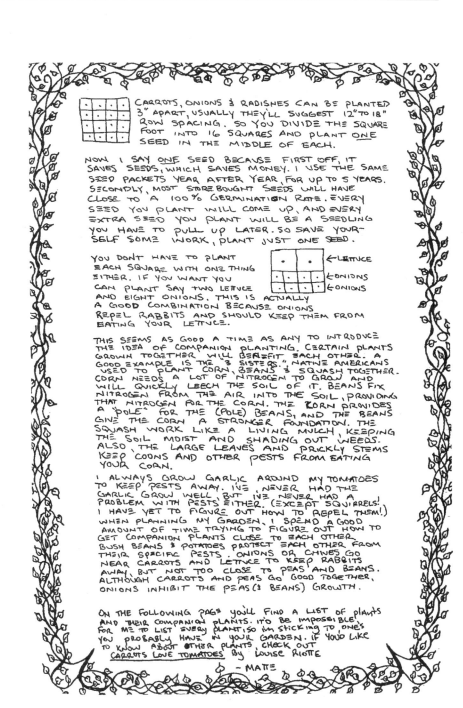

CARROTS, ONIONS & RADISHES CAN BE PLANTED 3" APART, USUALLY THEY'LL SUGGEST 12" TO 18" ROW SPACING. SO YOU DIVIDE THE SQUARE FOOT INTO 16 SQUARES AND PLANT ONE SEED IN THE MIDDLE OF EACH.

NOW I SAY ONE SEED BECAUSE FIRST OFF, IT SAVES SEEDS, WHICH SAVES MONEY. I USE THE SAME SEED PACKETS YEAR AFTER YEAR, FOR UP TO 5 YEARS. SECONDLY, MOST STORE BOUGHT SEEDS WILL HAVE CLOSE TO A 100% GERMINATION RATE. EVERY SEED YOU PLANT WILL COME UP, AND EVERY EXTRA SEED YOU PLANT WILL BE A SEEDLING YOU HAVE TO PULL UP LATER. SO SAVE YOUR-SELF SOME WORK, PLANT JUST ONE SEED.

YOU DON'T HAVE TO PLANT EACH SQUARE WITH ONE THING EITHER. IF YOU WANT YOU CAN PLANT SAY TWO LETTUCE AND EIGHT ONIONS. THIS IS ACTUALLY A GOOD COMBINATION BECAUSE ONIONS REPEL RABBITS AND SHOULD KEEP THEM FROM EATING YOUR LETTUCE.

THIS SEEMS AS GOOD A TIME AS ANY TO INTRODUCE THE IDEA OF COMPANION PLANTING. CERTAIN PLANTS GROWN TOGETHER WILL BENEFIT EACH OTHER. A GOOD EXAMPLE IS THE "3 SISTERS." NATIVE AMERICANS USED TO PLANT CORN, BEANS & SQUASH TOGETHER. CORN NEEDS A LOT OF NITROGEN TO GROW AND WILL QUICKLY LEECH THE SOIL OF IT. BEANS FIX NITROGEN FROM THE AIR INTO THE SOIL, PROVIDING THAT NITROGEN FOR THE CORN. THE CORN PROVIDES A "POLE" FOR THE (POLE) BEANS, AND THE BEANS GIVE THE CORN A STRONGER FOUNDATION. THE SQUASH WORK LIKE A LIVING MULCH, KEEPING THE SOIL MOIST AND SHADING OUT WEEDS. ALSO, THE LARGE LEAVES AND PRICKLY STEMS KEEP COONS AND OTHER PESTS FROM EATING YOUR CORN.

I ALWAYS GROW GARLIC AROUND MY TOMATOES TO KEEP PESTS AWAY. I'VE NEVER HAD THE GARLIC GROW WELL, BUT I'VE NEVER HAD A PROBLEM WITH PESTS EITHER. (EXCEPT SQUIRRELS! I HAVE YET TO FIGURE OUT HOW TO REPEL THEM!) WHEN PLANNING MY GARDEN, I SPEND A GOOD AMOUNT OF TIME TRYING TO FIGURE OUT HOW TO GET COMPANION PLANTS CLOSE TO EACH OTHER. BUSH BEANS & POTATOES PROTECT EACH OTHER FROM THEIR SPECIFIC PESTS. ONIONS OR CHIVES GO NEAR CARROTS AND LETTUCE TO KEEP RABBITS AWAY, BUT NOT TOO CLOSE TO PEAS AND BEANS. ALTHOUGH CARROTS AND PEAS GO GOOD TOGETHER, ONIONS INHIBIT THE PEAS (& BEANS) GROWTH.

ON THE FOLLOWING PAGE YOU'LL FIND A LIST OF PLANTS AND THEIR COMPANION PLANTS. IT'D BE IMPOSSIBLE FOR ME TO LIST EVERY PLANT, SO I'M STICKING TO ONE'S YOU PROBABLY HAVE IN YOUR GARDEN. IF YOU'D LIKE TO KNOW ABOUT OTHER PLANTS, CHECK OUT CARROTS LOVE TOMATOES BY LOUISE RIOTTE

— MATTE

Potatoes in a Barrel!!

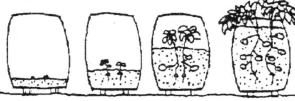

I got my hands on four plastic 50-gallon barrels.
I drilled drain holes in them, set them up on
blocks and planted spuds in them. Here's how: Cut
up potatoes which have started to sprout, leaving
an eye or more on each piece. Dry these out for
two days in a cool, dry room. Then plant in a
shallow layer of soil and compost in the bottom of
the barrel. As the potatoes grow up, add more soil
and compost. After they reach the top of the
barrel, I plant a couple of bush beans in each
barrel. The beans protect the potatoes against the
Colorado potato beetle, and the potatoes protect
the beans against the Mexican bean beetle. As soon
as the potatoes flower you can find little spuds
in the soil. When the whole plant dies back, kick
over the barrel for a bountiful harvest. I have
two barrels of red potatoes, one of white russet,
and one of Yukon gold.

AS PROMISED, HERE IS A GARDENING HINT.
I HAVEN'T ACTUALLY TRIED IT, BUT I'VE
SEEN PICTURES & WOW!! THAT'S A LOT
OF POTATOES! SORRY, DON'T HAVE MORE
THAN THIS. BUT I DO HAVE THE NAME
OF A BOOK THAT WAS SUGGESTED TO
ME, CARROTS LOVE TOMATOES — SECRETS
OF COMPANION GARDENING. by LOUISE RIOTTE

How to do a Germination Test

A germination test is incredibly easy to do. I just wet a paper towel, fold it in half, place about 20 seeds on one side (you can do as few as 5) and fold the other half over that. Then put that in a Ziploc or baggie (you can put more than one test in each bag) and put somewhere warm (like on top of the radiator.) After a few days, you can start taking them out and holding the still folded paper towel up to a light source to see if there are any sprouts. Give it another day or two after you see the first sprouts then open up and count how many seeds have sprouted. (18 out of 20=90% germination rate) If only half of your seeds sprout, it would be a good idea to sow them twice as thick. Large seeds like beans should be given plenty of room. If they are too close together, they may mold fouling up your test results.

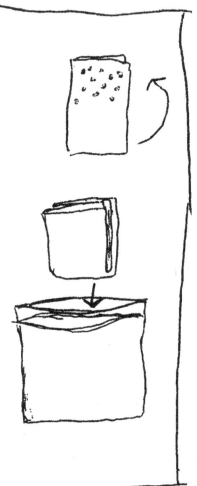

COMPOST

Lately I've been obsessed with two things - compost and homebrewing. There are a lot of similarities between the two. Both involve getting a few basic things together, things that can be scavenged or scrapped for; both involve getting a good recipe and having patience; both entail reusing stuff that other people might consider garbage, like empty bottles or kitchen scraps. And both are all about self-sufficiency and autonomy. Having more control in the cycle of what goes on all around you; what you produce, what you consume, what happens to your waste. It feels really good to make beer with natural ingredients, and re-use old bottles. It feels good to make sure my kitchen scraps get turned into compost, which geos into the garden to grow more vegetables, rather than going to the landfill. Closing the loop, being a part of the entire cycle, rather than feeling lost in a string of disconnected happenings. Seeing our efforts take shape and grow, like the micro-organisms that ferment the beer; like the micro-organisms that break down the compost.

Composting is easy, even in urban areas, and it's something just about everyone can and should do. A lot of what makes up land-fills is reusable and recyclable, and a lot of it is plant material that can be composted and used to provide nutrients for your plants. Composting makes sense especially if you live with lots of people and are cooking often, doing food not bombs, etc.

what goes in the compost?
leaves... poo? leaves...

An important part of composting is having the right recipe. Merrydeath suggests a three-part system: one part vegetable and kitchen scraps, one part horse, cow, or mule manure, and one part leaves, plant, and newspaper scraps. Not having manure readily available, I find a really easy recipe to follow is 50-50, kitchen scraps to dry leaves.

What you should NOT put in the compost are human, dog, and cat poop; meat products; excessive amounts of sugars; dairy by-products; large amounts of oil. The exception to dairy is egg-shells, which are beneficial. Diseased plants, like ones suffering from blight, should not be added to the compost because the disease can transfer to your plants.

Pay attention to what you're putting into the compost, watch how well different things break down. I find that breads tend to get moldy before they actually compost, and tea bags break down a lot slower than everything else on my pile. I've been told that non-organic orange peels are a bad idea, because they are so soaked in pesticides.

The C/N ratio:

Why such a fuss over ingredients? Well, compost organisms need a good proportion of carbon for energy and nitrogen for forming protein; called the C/N ratio. If there is too much carbon, plants break down slower and nitrogen - a key mineral for many of your

plants health - is depleted. If there is too much nitrogen your
compost will reek. A good way to keep a healthy ratio is to layer
the materials in your compost, alternating greens and browns. Green
are high in nitrogen, browns high in carbon.

GREENS

coffee grounds, cover crops, seaweed, grains, weeds, leaves,
hair (pet and human), fruit waste, veggie scraps, cow and horse
manure.

hay, nutshells, paper, straw, pine needles, veggie stalks
and seeds, sawdust, corncobs

BROWNS

water and air:

Two important aspects of your compost pile are wetness and
aeration. The pile should be moist, but not soggy - like a damp
sponge. Put it somewhere with good drainage, not in a pit where
water collects. A pallet floor is good for this, as well as for
aeration. The compost needs air-flow, so that everything will break
down properly. A pallet floor lets air in from underneath, and as
the compost breaks down, some will fall through - you can lift up
the entire bin to get the rich finished compost underneath.

Turn the pile often - this also helps with aeration. Don't
let kitchen scraps sit exposed, this will attract flies and rats.
It will also break down faster if incorporated into the pile, rather
than just flung on top. Keep a layer of leaves on top at all times,
and covering the pile with a tarp can help in a variety of ways:
keeping the pile warm in cold weather, helping to keep moisture in
if needed,, encouraging decomposition.

It feels so good to turn the pile and have it smell of that
musky rotting leaves smell, like in a forest after rain, and not
like a big pile of stinky rotting vegetables.

WORMS

Another good way to compost is using worms. This can be very
space efficient and quick. You can keep a worm bin under the kitchen
sink and they'll turn a couple square feet of scraps into good
compost within a few weeks, easy. You need to get special worms,
and there is a little bit of maintenance involved, but it can be
well worth the effort, especially if you don't have space outside
for a compost bin. The book Worms Eat My Garbage by Mary Appelhof
will tell you everything you need to know.

There are lots of different ways to compost, and most
libraries have books full of information about it. My friend
Sarah and I built a really simple compost bin that works great
at my house, using pallets and some chicken wire. I wanted it
to have doors and a hinged top, but it's just fine without that
stuff.

THE DOUBLE BIN WE HAVE AT MY HOUSE. WORKS GREAT!

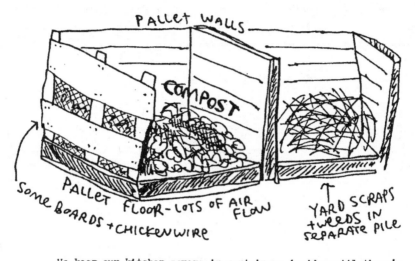

PALLET WALLS

COMPOST

SOME BOARDS + CHICKENWIRE
PALLET FLOOR - LOTS OF AIR FLOW

YARD SCRAPS + WEEDS IN SEPARATE PILE

We keep our kitchen scraps in containers inside until there's a good amount, and then take it out the pile, throw on some leaves, and turn it all together, mix it up, making sure that food isn't left exposed. YOU CAN ALSO KEEP KITCHEN SCRAPS IN THE FREEZER TO KEEP BUGS AWAY AND PREVENT MOLD.

Information from Merrydeath's zine Crude Noise, and the book Backyard Composting, as well as my own experimentation and experience (and my housemates, who are almost as compost crazed as I am).

I'M SUCH A DORK ABOUT THIS STUFF - WHENEVER I GET BACK HOME, ONE OF THE FIRST THINGS I DO IS CHECK ON THE WORMS, THE COMPOST. IT'S SO SATISFYING.

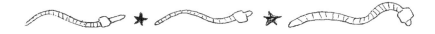

Time to Feed the Worms

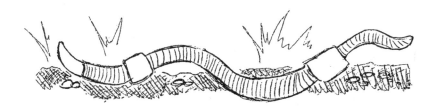

by Martha Riecks
Here Be Dragons
Mike Q Roth, Eric eds.

Until a few months ago, I had no clue about what earthworms did. I would almost guarantee I had never even thought about it until one day in geology class. Surprisingly, worms are nature's fertilizer and the key to usable soil. Their burrowing loosens soil while providing it with necessary oxygen. As worms move through the soil, they consume decaying vegetable matter. The resulting excretions, called castings, are full of nitrogen and other nutrients that are the key to healthy soil that plants will thrive in.

Just a few days later, Chris and Q stumbled along the same facts while continuing their search to decrease the amount of trash created by the Eco-crew. Worms eat garbage. Thus, you have less trash to add to landfill piles and compost to mix into soil. And all this magic takes place underneath the kitchen sink. Yet could we deal with this new pet? Not that we'd have to walk or bathe the worms, but we haven't completely mastered feeding ourselves regularly, much less being responsible for feeding 1,000 lives with our table scraps. But the cru-

cial question was would it smell? Would the worms make friends with the roaches and encourage them to take up residence under our sink? And how were we to remember all the names?

There was only one way to find out, so we tried it! Setting it up sounds rather tedious and it was... find a bin... find a drill... find worms. But once you've done all that, it gets really really easy.

The bin can be either wood or plastic, between 8 and 12 inches deep. You need one square foot of surface area available for every pound of compostable garbage produced by the household in one week. We were hoping to find a discarded dresser drawer to use, but we ended up buying one of those plastic storage boxes that fits under the bed. There are several manufactured worm bins available, but they all looked very similar to the heavy-duty plastic utility boxes you can buy at your local discount mega-shop for about 1/2 the price.

At least 8 small holes should be drilled in the bottom of the container for drainage (you will need more if you use a plastic container since it will not absorb water like a wooden bin can). Elevate it slightly to allow for drainage and place something underneath it to catch the runoff. We took the lid from the storage box (upper side down), placed small flower pots on it, and set the worm bin on top of these.

The container you choose for a bin helps to determine where to place it. Wood is better insulated and will block light, so it works well for colder areas and bright rooms while translucent plastic bins must kept in a dark area. Basements are highly recommended but many people just keep the bins on their countertop. We put ours in a cabinet to keep the bin out of the way, but this is sometimes a pain when I go to add the garbage, maneuvering it out and back in, but it keeps it away from the cat.

Fill the bin a little less than three-fourths full with shredded newspaper, peat moss, dead plants, crumbled fall leaves, aged manure, or compost. We used a mixture of these, figuring worms like variety just like we do (and it gives them more nutrients). The worms will need a little bit of gritty soil or sand to help with digestion. Don't pack the bedding tightly since air pockets will help to prevent odors.

Now that you have a nice home for the worms, you must acquire them. You do not want dew worms or nightcrawlers; they don't compost as well and will probably not survive. You want *Eisenia foetida*, that's redworms, red wrigglers, brandlings or manure worms. Planning to purchase them at a live bait store if you live in the city does not work! (Trust me, we tried.) It will only delay the final step in the creation of your worm bin.

The most efficient way to order them is by mail. Many suppliers can be found on the Internet. They've heard of this before and will send you the right worms. We ordered our new roommates from the Kazarie Worm Farm. Or you could check in your area to see if there is a worm farm or anybody who already worm composts and has worms to spare.

How many worms you will need varies. One book said a 1:1 ratio is best (one pound of garbage per day for one pound of worms) while a web page recommends a 1:2 ratio (one pound of garbage per day for two pounds of worms). We decided to get 1 pound of worms (approximately 1,000 critters), figuring that if there was too much garbage for the worms to eat, we just wouldn't put it all in. The worms also multiply so if you didn't get enough to start with, don't worry, just give them a little time.

DEALIN' IN WIGGLERS

Kazarie Worm Farm " Quality Redworms and Castings"

Dan Warco, Owner
7370 SE 56th Terrace
Trenton, FL 32693
352-463-7823
Fax: 352-463-3944
www.afn.org/~Kazarie
email: Kazarie@afn.org

1-4 pounds...$14.50 per pound

Flowerfield Enterprise
Mary Appelhof, Owner
10332 Shaver Rd
Kalamazoo, MI 49024
616-327-0108
Fax: 616-327-7009
www.wormwoman.com

Worm-a-Way Worm Bin
(Price includes worms and a copy of Worms eat my Garbage)
Small (1-3 lbs per week) $76.00
Large (3-5 lbs per week) $89.00
1 pound of worms $24.00
2 pounds of worms $41.00

Let's Get Growing
Educational Supply Company
800-408-1868
letsgetgrowing.com/pages/worms.html

Wonder Worm Kit $45.00
(includes worms)
1 pound of worms $25.00
2 pounds of worms $35.00

WHAT TO FEED YOUR WORMS

Pro-active	De-active
Fruit (including peels)	Dairy Products
Any vegetable matter	Meat Products
Tea Bags (take out the staples)	Oils, Greases, and Fat
Coffee Grounds (including filter)	Peanut Butter
Pasta	Wood Chips
Bread	Salt
Cereals	Bones
Eggshells (crushed)	Vinegar

(Traces of salad dressing on lettuce are alright, just don't glob it in)

THIS DOESN'T SEEM TO BE WORKING...

The worms are crawling out of the bedding: They are declaring that the bin conditions are wrong for them. Is the moisture level right? If the soil is too wet, check the drainage holes for clogs. Try leaving the cover off for a little bit to see if the excess water will evaporate. Or you might need to drill more holes (just dump the bin out on plastic and refill after drilling) to improve drainage.

If the moisture level is not the problem, then it is likely the worms find the bin too acidic. This can be aggravated by the addition of orange peels and other acidic wastes. Try adding a little garden lime, some crushed eggshells, or sprinkling baking soda to counteract the acidity.
It's beginning to look like a Fruit Fly bin. Make sure that your garbage is properly buried and that you are putting the cover back on the bin. (if you constantly leave it off for evaporation as mentioned above, then you need to drill more holes). If none of this helps; try finding a new location near lots of spiders or inside an enclosed area (like a cabinet).
It just stinks. This happens if you put in too much waste (or too much in one area) and the worms can't digest it before it starts rotting. Limit the amount of food waste you are putting in. If the problem persists, try giving the bin a good stirring to allow more air in and provide the bin more ventilation. Or the bin could be waterlogged; check the drainage holes for clogs or drill more.

A really strong, chemically smell can be caused by composting bacteria that have developed in the bin. I try to just bury whatever is really smelly although I have noticed that this is often an indicator that your bin is approaching harvest point.

The worms need the contents of the bin to be damped. We use a trigger sprayer to gently mist the bedding until it has the moisture of a well-rung out sponge. Do not let the soil get too wet or your new pets will drown. (This is why you drilled drainage holes.) Lay a piece of burlap or a plastic garbage bag over the top of the bin to provide insulation and retain moisture. Using a tight cover will suffocate the worms— they need oxygen to breathe! If you want to use a sturdier cover, cut lots of openings in it for ventilation.

From here, it gets easier. Just take your organic garbage, gently dig a small hole, place the garbage in it, and cover it with bedding (try to space your burial spots around the bin). The worms will not need everything pureed, but they cannot compost an entire whole carrot. Make sure you break larger chunks before burying it. Check the moisture of the entire mixture and mist if needed. That's all. Don't panic if you don't feed them something everyday, they'll have plenty to decompose.

After about two and a half months most of the original bedding will have disappeared. It will have been replaced by dark brown castings, a nutrient-rich compost that your flower beds will love. But the worms won't, you must provide them new bedding to decompose. The fastest way to do this is to shove as much of the finished compost that you can to one side of the bin, and fill in the empty side with a mixture of new bedding materials and compost. Bury your garbage here. The worms will figure out they want to be on this side of the bin, and you should be able to gradually remove the finished compost as you need it (adding a little more new bedding each time you do so).

If you want all the compost or are very bored one day, you can simply dump out the entire worm bin (preferably on a plastic sheet). Refill the bin with bedding mixed with a small amount of compost. Then go through the compost on the sheet to pick out the worms and put them back into their bin. (Don't panic if you find tiny oval shaped things. You are probably looking at the worm cocoons that contain baby worms. Put these all in the bin too, unless you need severe worm population control.) If you don't need all of the compost, it can be stored in plastic bags.

The compost can be mixed in with potting soil, spread on the top of soil in pots, used as an outdoor mulch, or worked into soil. Two months ago this was garbage— now it's fertilizer. Just the end result of this useful little fellow's dietary cycle. Worms...they're not the most exciting pet in the world, but what they can do.

sprouts are good ✳✳✳✳

HOW TO SPROUT 1·2·3 + TIPS!

Sprouts are houseplants you can eat! They are an excellent source of vitamins and minerals, and are both ECONOMICAL and ECOLOGICAL!

three steps to sprouting food

#1 Pour in seed. Cover with more than 2x the water (tap).

SOAK OVERnight...

#2

Rinse 'til water runs clear. DRAIN WELL! Repeat every morn. + eve. for 3 days...

EASY · FUN

#3 Between rinses

KEEP SPROUTS AWAY FROM LIGHT. COVER WITH A → DISH CLOTH

air vent!

EAT

MORE TIPS

Best Fresh!

SPROUTS VEGAN AVOCADO

REFRIGERATE LEFTOVERS

cheese

EGGS

SPROUTS

LEFTOVERS

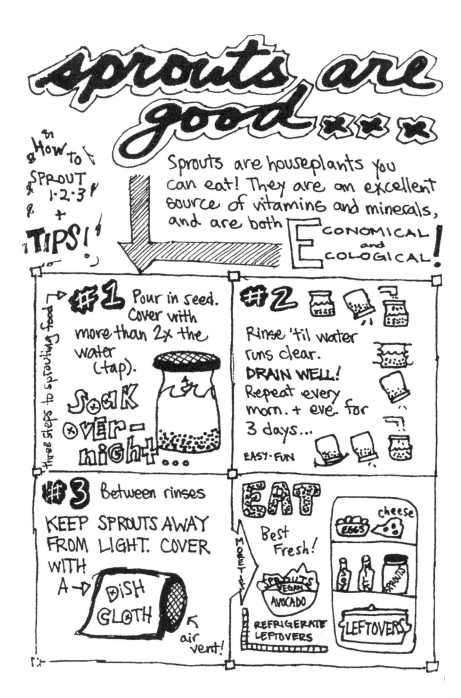

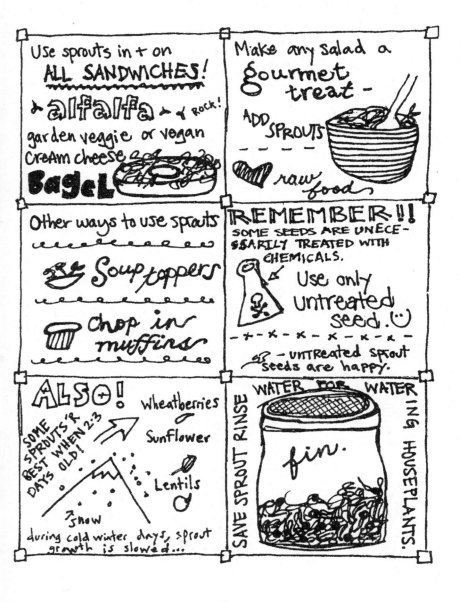

Use sprouts in + on ALL SANDWICHES!
alfalfa ~ rock!
garden veggie or vegan cream cheese
Bagel

Make any salad a gourmet treat –
ADD SPROUTS
raw food

Other ways to use sprouts
Soup toppers
Chop in muffins

REMEMBER!!
SOME SEEDS ARE UNECESSARILY TREATED WITH CHEMICALS.
Use only untreated seed. :)
– untreated sprout seeds are happy.

ALSO!
SOME SPROUTS 'R BEST WHEN 2-3 DAYS OLD!
Wheatberries
Sunflower
Lentils
snow
during cold winter days, sprout growth is slowed...

SAVE SPROUT RINSE WATER FOR WATERING HOUSEPLANTS.
fin.

Solar Dehydrating EDIBLE WILD ONIONS

LAST SUMMER I NOTICED ALL THESE DARK GREEN THINGS GROWING ALL OVER THE PLACE THAT LOOKED LIKE CHIVES. ONE DAY I PLUCKED A PIECE OFF OF ONE & STUCK IT IN MY MOUTH. IT TASTED ONIONY/GARLICKY. "WOW" I THOUGHT TO MYSELF, "EDIBLE WILD ONIONS, & THEY'RE EVERY-WHERE!" SO THIS YEAR, AFTER WINTER WENT AWAY I NOTICED THEM SPROUTING UP AGAIN ALL OVER THE PLACE. SO I HEADED OUT WITH A BUCKET & SOME SCISSORS & SNIPPED UP EVERYONE I CAME ACROSS UNTIL MY BUCKET WAS FULL. WHEN I GOT HOME I RINSED THEM OFF & CHOPPED THEM UP INTO LITTLE PIECES. I SPREAD THEM OUT ON A SCREEN FROM A WINDOW & LAID THEM OUT THE NEXT DAY ON TOP OF JENNY'S CAR IN THE SUN. IT WAS A 97° DAY & THE ADDED HEAT REFLECTED OFF THE CAR PROB-ABLY MADE IT HOTTER. OVER THE COURSE OF THE DAY THE HEAT ALONG WITH A SLIGHT BREEZE TOGETHER TOTALLY DRIED OUT THE ONIONS LEAVING THEM IN A PRESERVED STATE READY TO BE USED IN COOKING AT A LATER DATE.

Insulative Cooking
Julie Summers

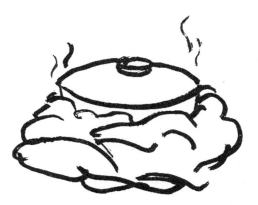

Insulative cooking is also known as "hay box" cooking because you can use hay to insulate with. However, hay is only one of many materials that insulate. Towels, blankets, sleeping bags, and clothes are other possibilities. The food is cooked over a flame, as usual, by bringing to a boil and simmering. However, with this method, the simmering time can be cut by half or more. Then the pot is covered with your insulation, and the heat it retains finishes the cooking. Nest the pot in the insulation so there are no large air spaces around it. Add insulation until there are four or more inches of it all around the pot. When using this method for short grain brown rice, I bring the water and rice to a boil, simmer seven minutes, then insulate about an hour and it's ready to eat. I do practically all my cooking this way now.

How to Season a Cast Iron Skillet

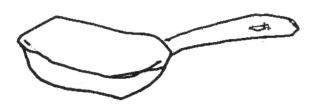

This may sound a bit trivial, but a good, blackened, cast iron skillet can be an indispensable part of your kitchen. It can be used several times a day, and you can bake, fry, saute, brown, or scramble anything in it. Some traditionalists say lard must be used, but here's an alternative technique. Play some black metal while waiting (i.e. the Sacramentum, *Thy Black Destiny* lp).

1. Wash the skillet with hot, soapy water and a stiff brush. Rinse and dry completely.

2. Oil the skillet inside and out with melted, solid vegetable oil shortening.

3. Turn upside down on the top rack of a preheated, 350° oven.

4. Put aluminum foil on the bottom rack to catch excess drippings.

5. Bake the skillet for 1 hour at 350.°

6. Let the skillet cool slowly in the oven.

7. Store, uncovered, in a dry place when cooled. Use as needed.

EGG REPLACER

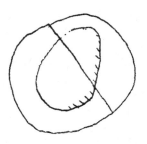

In baking, eggs are traditionally used as a sort of binder, basically to hold all the stuff together. While eggs do work well for this purpose, some of us don't eat eggs (or any other animal products), so we need an alternative to replace eggs in our baked goods. I've found that just a simple mixture of corn starch and a little water mixed together make a good egg replacer. Also, bananas do a pretty good job as an egg stand-in. This is a recipe for egg replacer from the zine, *Grandma Ida*, by Angie, G.:

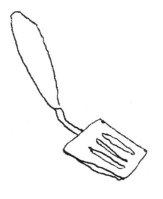

½ tsp potato starch
½ tsp corn starch
½ tsp tapioca flour
5 tsp water
1 tsp oil

Angie says, "you can substitute more corn starch for the potato starch, normal flour for the tapioca flour, and more water for the oil, if you want or need to. Mix it all together before you use it. This equals one egg."

DON'T GET KNOCKED OUT BY A CREAM PUFF

Recently in a small bakery's dumpster, I found some gourmet croissants (neatly packaged in their original bag). They were filled with cheese, ham, turkey, or vegetables (all tremendously more perishable than plain bread, rolls, or sweet pastries), which prompted me to review my food poisoning notes -- taken from Ptomaine, by Stewart Brooks (Barnes '74), and "You Can Avoid Food Poisoning" by Susan Zarrow (Prevention , April 1986).

In one type of food poisoning, bacteria produce toxins in the food before it is eaten (eg, botulism and staph). In the other type, bacteria infect you, after the food is eaten (eg, salmonella).

Most bacteria do not grow in food when its internal temperature is under 40°F or over 150°F, hence the importance of keeping food cold, or hot.

Botulism spores germinate when conditions are right, especially when there is a lack of oxygen -- which can happen in the can, and "in foods (particularly fish) where certain biochemical agents 'absorb' oxygen", says Brooks. The botulism toxin is destroyed by heat. Zarrow says a few minutes boiling is enough; elsewhere I've read 25 minutes. I assume bigger pieces of food take longer to heat all the way thru. (To kill botulism spores, to make canned food ←temperatures above boiling are required -- hence the need for pressure canning.) store without becoming poisonous.

Nearly all cases of staph poisoning can be traced to food handlers. (I assume via pussy sores. I'm not sure about nasal secretions or saliva one medical text says 30-40% of normal people carry staph bacteria in their nostrils, but some pathogens are transmitted that way. It's best if food handlers refrain from smoking (because cigarettes can transmit saliva to the hands), or touching their noses, mouths, or crotches -- or if they do, as when wiping themselves after defecating, they wash their hands.)

Most staph poisonings are caused by cream and custard fillings; followed by ham and cheddar cheese; also milk, creamed tuna, and ice cream. Heating the food will kill staph bacteria but will not destroy staph toxins already produced. Keep them from being produced, by keeping food cold (under 40°F) or hot (over 150°F). Symptoms of staph poisoning are vomitting and diarrhea, which develop one to six hours after eating contaminated food.

Salmonella is passed in feces of people or animal carriers. Any type of food or drink can be contaminated. 0.2% of people are asymptomatic carriers. Salmonella is killed by heat -- Brooks says a few minutes at 140°F; Zarrow says when the food reaches 165°F internally. (Boiling is 212°F at sea level.) After eating contaminated food, a couple of days may pass before the bacteria multiply enough to cause symptoms, such as diarrhea. Cross contamination can be a problem, eg, cutting raw chicken and then touching salad ingredients with fingers, knife, or cutting board. The chicken gets sterilized by cooking, but the salad, eaten raw, remains infected. contaminated

Food which supports rapid growth of bacteria includes all kinds of meat, eggs, milk and milk products, cooked vegetables; and foods containing these diseases", says Zarrow. "You put an awful lot of faith in people when you eat in a restaurant ", says University of MN microbiology professor, Dr. Zottola.
"Restaurants are associated with about half of all outbreaks of foodborne

Zarrow says moldy bread and other baked goods should be discarded entirely, but okay to eat hard-block cheese, hard salami and smoked turkey after cutting away at least an inch beyond the moldy spot.

Back to the croissants: adequate heating would destroy any salmonella, as well as any staph bacteria, but not staph toxin. Thus, after heating, I would eat only a small amount , and wait 1-6 hours. If no symptoms occurred I would assume the food was okay to eat more of. I would keep the food cold while waiting, because even after heating, airborne bacteria could land on the food, and grow if conditions were right.

THE MINIMUM SOLAR BOX COOKER

A DESIGN YOU CAN BUILD IN 2-4 HOURS FOR ALMOST NOTHING

1. Insulation is not essential in the walls — a foiled airspace is all that is necessary.

2. Aluminum foil can be reduced to just one layer (though a layer on the inside of each box makes a hotter oven).

3. The airspace between the walls can be very small. The smallest airspace we've tested is one inch, but we suspect that even less would work.

4. Almost any size oven will cook. In general, larger ovens get hotter. But the limiting factor is still the ratio between the mass of the food and the size of the oven (we cooked a liter of beets in late-September in Seattle using an oven with an opening only 10" x 14" (25cm x 35cm).

5. Our experience shows that a double layer of plastic film works at least as well as a single sheet of glass.

6. Shallower ovens cook better since they have less wall area through which to lose heat. It's best for the inside of the oven to be just slightly taller than the biggest pot you plan to use.

WHAT YOU WILL NEED

Two cardboard boxes, homemade, scavenged, or bought. Almost any size will work. The proportion between the two boxes is not critical. We would suggest that you use an inner box that is at least 15" x 15" (38cm x 38cm). The outer box should be larger all around, but it doesn't matter how much bigger as long as there is an inch (2.5cm) or more of an airspace between the two boxes. Also note that the distance between the two boxes does not have to be equal all the way around. Thus, with rectangular boxes, the long sides might have a bigger airspace than the short sides or visa versa.

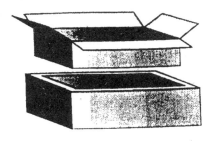

Figure 1

One sheet of cardboard to make the lid. This piece must be at least 3" (7.5cm) larger all the way around than the top of the finished cooker.

One small roll of aluminum foil.

One small jar of black tempera paint, or black soot from clear wood.

At least 8 ounces of white glue or wheat paste.

One Reynolds® Oven Cooking Bag (or sheet of glass). These are available in almost all supermarkets in the U.S. They are rated for 400° F (204.4 C) so they are perfect for solar cooking. They are not UV resistant; thus they will become more brittle and opaque over time and may need to be replaced periodically. (Barbara Kerr has experimented with the kitchen grade plastic wraps. Glad Wrap® is the only kitchen grade plastic film recommended at this time due to the chemical composition of all others investigated so far. Although it is not rated for the temperatures produced in solar ovens, it seems to work as glazing as long as the opening is not wider than the plastic. If the opening is wider than the plastic, sometimes the inherent cling will join two pieces. Some of these plastics, such as Saran Wrap® and the Reynolds Wraps® are made of Polyvinyline Chloride and there are still questions about their safety around food at solar box cooker temperatures).

CONSTRUCTION

BUILDING THE BASE

Fold the top flaps closed on the outer box and set the inner box on top and trace a line around it onto the top of the outer box. Remove the inner box and cut along this line to form a hole in the top of the outer box (Figure 1).

Decide how deep you want your oven to be (about 1" or 2.5cm bigger than your largest pot and at least 1" shorter than the outer box) and slit the corners of the inner box down to that height. Fold each side down forming extended flaps (Figure 2). Folding is smoother if you first draw a firm line from the end of one cut to the other where the folds are to go.

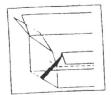

Figure 2

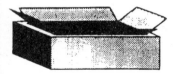

Figure 3

Glue foil to the inside of both boxes and also to the inside of the remaining top flaps of the outer box. Don't waste your time being neat on the outer box, since it will never be seen, nor will it experience any wear. The inner box will be visible even after assembly, so if it matters to you, you might want to take more time here. Glue the top flaps closed on the outer box.

Place some wads of crumpled newspaper into the outer box so that when you set the inner box down inside the hole in the outer box, the flaps on the inner box just touch the top of the outer box (Figure 3). Glue these flaps onto the top of the outer box. Trim the excess flap length to be even with the perimeter of the outer box. The base is now finished.

BUILDING THE LID

Take the large sheet of cardboard and lay it on top of the base. Trace its outline and then cut and fold down the edges to form a lip of about 3" (7.5cm). Fold the corners around and glue (Figure 4). Orient the corrugations so that they go from left to right as you face the oven so that later the prop may be inserted into the corrugations (Figure 6). One trick you can use to make the lid fit well is to lay the pencil or pen against the side of the box when marking (Figure 5).

To make the reflector flap, draw a line on the lid, forming a rectangle the same size as the oven opening. Cut around three sides and fold the

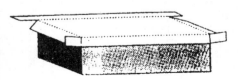

Figure 4

resulting flap up forming the reflector (Figure 6), and appy foil to the flap on the inside.

To make a prop bend a 12" (30cm) piece of hanger wire as indicated in Figure 6. This can then be inserted into the corrugations as shown.

Next, turn the lid upside-down and glue the oven bag (or other glazing material) in place. We have had great success using the turkey size oven bag (19" x 23 1/2", 47.5cm x 58.5cm) applied as is, i.e. without opening it up. This makes a double layer of plastic. The two layers tend to separate from each other to form an airspace as the oven cooks. When using this method, it is important to also

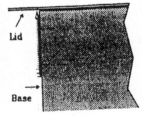

Lid

Base

glue the bag closed on its open end. This stops water vapor from entering the bag and condensing. Alternately you can cut any size oven bag open to form a flat sheet large enough to cover the oven opening.

Finally, to make the drip pan, cut a piece of cardboard, the same size as the bottom of the interior of the oven and apply foil to one side. Paint this foiled side black and allow it to dry. Put this in the oven (black side up) and place

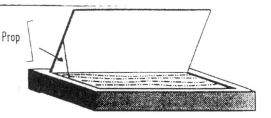

Prop

Figure 6

IMPROVING EFFICIENCY

The oven you have built should cook fine during most of the solar season. If you would like to improve the efficiency to be able to cook on more marginal days, you can modify your oven in any or all of the following ways:

1. Make pieces of foiled cardboard the same size as the oven sides and place these in the wall spaces.

2. Make a new reflector the size of the entire lid.

3. Make the drip pan using aluminum flashing and elevate this off the bottom of the oven slightly with small cardboard strips.

SPEEDY SOLAR CHOCOLATE CAKE

This cake can be mixed in the pan you're going to cook it in.

> 1 1/2 cups sifted flour
> 3 tablespoons cocoa
> 1 teaspoon baking soda
> 1 cup sugar
> 1/2 teaspoon salt
> 5 tablespoons cooking oil
> 1 tablespoon vinegar
> 1 teaspoon vanilla
> 1 cup cold water

Put your sifted flour back in the sifter; add the cocoa, baking powder, sugar, and salt. Sift the ingredients into an oiled 9" square pan. Make three grooves, or holes, in the dry mixture. Into one, pour the oil; into the next, the vinegar; into the next, the vanilla. Pour the cold water over it all. Mix until it's smooth and you can't see the flour. Bake at 300° for 45 minutes. Serves 6.

FRENCH-ITALIAN BREAD

> 1 package active dry yeast
> 1 cup warm water (110°F)
> 1 1/2 teaspoons sugar
> 1 teaspoon salt
> 2 - 3 cups flour
> 1/4 cup corn meal

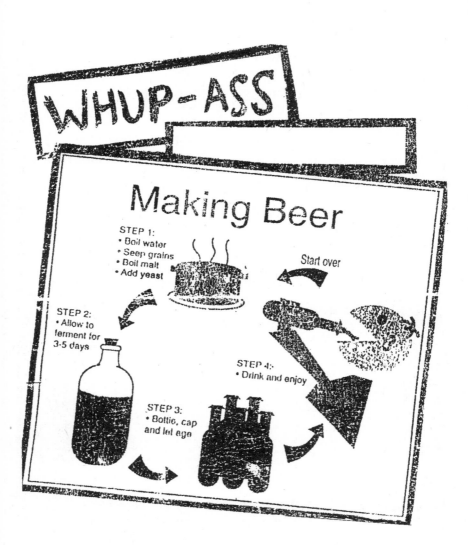

WHUP-ASS

Making Beer

STEP 1:
• Boil water
• Seep grains
• Boil malt
• Add yeast

Start over

STEP 2:
• Allow to
ferment for
3-5 days

STEP 4:
• Drink and enjoy

STEP 3:
• Bottle, cap
and let age

Making Beer

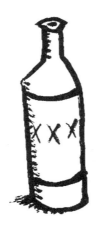

Making Beer is about as hard as making coffee. There are innumerable books out there about how to do it (*The New Complete Joy of Homebrewing* by Charlie Papazian, for example). They explain what flavors the hops and malts and other adjuncts bring to the beer. There are also a lot of books that try to make the whole thing sound complex and intimidating. Fuck that! "Beer Brewing Equipment and Supplies" is the heading for beer supply stores in the Portland Yellow Pages; it's probably something similar in your town. You should have about $50 in your pocket for start up costs (which isn't too bad when you consider that a case of beer can cost about $15).

Okay, so beer is made up of 4 ingredients: hops, barley, water, and yeast. Sure you can throw in other things; that's why there are a million beer-making books. The last batch of beer I made was about a week ago so I'll just give you that recipe and tell you what I did.

Out of the cupboard comes a big pot, cheese cloth, 5 gallon plastic bucket, carboy (large plastic or glass container that looks like those bottles on water coolers), thermometer, siphoning tube, fermentation lock, rubber stopper, ½ lb. honey malt (grain), 1 ½ lbs. pale malt (grain), 7 lbs. pale malt extract (syrup), 1 oz. Northern Brewers hops, 1 oz. Yakima Kent Golding hops, and one package of Edme yeast. I use a combo of extract and grains for the malt, but you can make all-grain or you can make all-extract!

Sanitizing? I use iodine or some other nontoxic no-rinse sanitizer. Wash out your stuff before you use it. I only sanitize the plastic bucket, carboy, siphoning tube, and bottles.

So, you fill your pot up about halfway with water and your grain. While waiting for it to boil put a bunch of water in your fridge and freezer for later and put the hops in the cheesecloth. Put aside about ½ oz. of hops to be your finishing hops (which means you add them at the very end), and bunch up the rest of them in about 3 cheesecloth bags (like tea!). Once the water and grains come to a boil (this is where it's called a "wort"), strain out the grain. Put the wort back on the stove and add the malt extract and the first hops (what, in my case, was the 1 ½ oz.)

At this point you should keep the wort simmering and keep stirring it. If it boils over it's a pain in the ass to clean up, so keep a glass of cold water next to the stove. You'll pour it into the pot if it starts to boil over. Now wait. About 40 minutes later add the finishing hops. 2 minutes later dump this wort into the plastic bucket through a strainer. Add the ice and cold water you made earlier to lower the wort temperature to about 78 degrees and buck up the volume to 5 gallons. Add the yeast. Yeast usually takes about 10 minutes to activate (you can read the directions while waiting). Siphon your raw beer into the carboy. Put the stopper and fermentation lock on, and clean up your mess.

Keep an eye on the fermentation lock. It should be moving, releasing a gas byproduct which proves the yeast is eating the sugar and producing alcohol. This is the time to play music for your beer – Sewer Trout, Poison Idea, or any of those songs-about-drinking comps.

About a week after you've made the beer the fermentation cap won't move anymore and it's time to bottle. Siphon the beer from the carboy into the bucket. In the bucket put ¾ cup of corn sugar, then siphon it into bottles. Cap them, wait about a month, and you've got beer! Now, just like Hippycore says, "Drink up and be fuckin' stoked!"

HOMEMADE ROOT BEER

Adapted from an article submitted for inclusion n the How2 Zine, by an author whose name has been lost. Also, based on my own personal experience trying this myself.

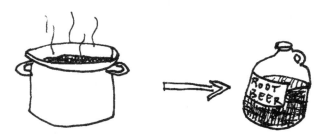

There's basically 2 ways to make root beer. You can use store-bought root beer extract, or you can use the actual real roots and herbs for flavor. They taste different depending which way you do it, but both are good. Of course, for the sake of DIY, I'm obligated to endorse the real roots and herbs over any store-bought concoction.

SUPPLIES

Either way you do it, you'll still need the same supplies to make root beer. You'll need a big pot, maybe like 2 – 5 gallons, depending how much root beer you want to make. You'll need containers that are airtight to store your root beer in (wine jugs, soda bottles, a bucket with a lid). You can reuse bottles that previously had other stuff in them, just be sure to clean them out really good. You're also going to need a straining device of some sort. You can get straining cloths and bags from homebrewing suppliers, or you can use cheesecloth (which you can get at hardware stores), or even an old t-shirt. A colander can work too, though sometimes the holes on colanders are a little too big and let too much debris through.

MAIN INGREDIENTS

Depending how much root beer you want to make, you'll need to adjust these measurements accordingly. Aside from the flavoring, which you get from the herbs, the basic ingredients of root beer are water, sweetener, and yeast. If you were going to make one gallon of root beer then you would need one gallon of water, 1 – 3 cups of sweetener, and about ¼ tsp of yeast. More sweetener makes a sweeter root beer, but less will allow the natural flavors of the roots and herbs to be more powerful. It's up to your own individual preference. Sugar is the obvious choice for sweetener, but you can also use honey, molasses, unrefined sugars, or any mixture of these. Yeast is available from homebrewing suppliers. It's what makes the root beer carbonated. You can also use bread yeast from the grocery store, but it tends to make the root beer more acidic, whereas the stuff from the homebrewing suppliers is intended specifically for brewing, so it's better.

HERBS

You can use many different herbs to flavor your root beer in different ways. You can get most of these from health food stores or homebrewing suppliers. Though there are many to choose from, the main one you'll need is sassafras root bark, or if you want to do it the less fun way, then you can just use root beer extract. You can actually harvest your own sassafras root if you live in areas where it grows. I think it's pretty plentiful in the southeast US.

Depending on your personal tastes you may also want to try adding some of these other herbs. Some good ones are: wintergreen, sasparilla, hops, crushed juniper berries, dandelion root, small pieces of licorice root or anise seed, cherry bark, vanilla beans, burdock, ginger.

INSTRUCTIONS

If you're just using extract, and not any herbs, pour the water into your pot then add the extract and your sweetener. Warm this up in the pot, but don't bring it all the way to a boil.

If you're using herbs, not extract, you basically want to make a big batch of tea with them to start off. Put them in the pot along with your water and boil them for half an hour to an hour. The goal is to cook as much of the flavoring out of the roots and into the water. It should turn dark and start to smell really good. After you've sufficiently cooked them, turn off the heat, and strain the herbs out of the water, then pour the water back into your pot. Add your sweetener, and stir.

Let this concoction cool down to a lukewarm temperature. Once it has cooled down it's time to add the yeast. The yeast is what will make your root beer carbonated. The yeast eat the sugars and give off carbonation as a byproduct, which, in turn, makes your root beer bubbly.

BOTTLING

As soon as you add the yeast to your root beer, it's time to bottle it. You may want to use a funnel to pour it into your bottle. Cap your bottle off and make sure it's sealed real good so no carbonation can escape. Let it sit for about half a day to a full day. This should be long enough to develop some good carbonation in your root beer. You may need to let out some of the air from your bottle every now and then just to make sure it doesn't build up too much pressure and explode.

Another way to avoid your bottle exploding from the build up of carbonation is to use an "airlock." You can get these from homebrewing suppliers. They come in different shapes, but the basic idea is that they allow excess air to escape, but don't let any air back into the bottle. You can also create your own airlock with a balloon. Just stretch the lip of a balloon over the top of your bottle. The balloon will fill with excess carbonation. You can just let air out of the balloon every few hours or so.

After 12 hours, your root beer should be ready to drink. Stick it in the refrigerator. This will essentially stop the yeast from producing any more carbonation. Now your root beer is done. Drink up!

HOW TO MAKE WINE

I've been making wine at home for many years. I seem to constantly make small changes in the process in an effort to make it simpler and quicker. The way I do it these days is to use a 64 ounce bottle of grape juice, which is the cheapest generic grape juice I find in the supermarket, to make 3 gallons of wine at a time. Here's the way I do it:

Equipment: 3 1-gallon glass jugs, 3-quart pan, 2 2-cup measuring cups, large funnel, drinking glass, 2 large spoons, 1/3 cup measuring cup, 3 small plastic bags, 6 large rubber bands.

Supplies: 64 ounce bottle of grape juice, packet of active dry bread yeast, sugar, water.

Procedure:
   1. Put a little sugar in the glass. Add some warm water, 1/2 cup more or less. Add the yeast and stir it occasionally while doing the following steps.
   2. Measure out 4 cups of sugar and pour it into the 3-quart pan. (I use 2 measuring cups so I can keep one dry for measuring sugar, and one wet for measuring grape juice.)
   3. Measure out 1/3 of the grape juice (that's 21 1/3 fluid ounces, which equals about 1 2/3 cup plus 1 cup) and pour it onto the sugar in the pan.

4. Mix with the spoon to dissolve the sugar into a slurry, then pour it thru the funnel into one of the gallon jugs. Add some water to the pan and slosh it around to dissolve the remaining sugar and add that to the jug.

5. Repeat steps 2, 3, and 4 to put sugar and grape juice into the other 2 jugs.

6. Pour yeast solution into the wet measuring cup. Add water to bring it up to 1 cup. Stir to mix. Use the 1/3 cup measuring cup to put 1/3 cup of this yeast solution thru the funnel into each of the gallon jugs.

7. Add water to bring the level up to the shoulders of the jugs.

8. Put a clean, small plastic bag over the top of each jug to serve as an airlock (to allow CO_2 to escape, but not allow air (oxygen) to get in). Fasten it on by wrapping 2 large rubber bands around the neck of the jug. (The 2nd rubber band is for insurance in case one breaks.)

9. The mixture may foam up when the yeast starts working. That's why I fill only to the shoulder at first, to leave room for the foam, so it doesn't foam out of the top and make a mess. After a couple days, when the foam has died down, mix by swirling each jug around to put into solution the sugar that has settled to the bottom of the jug.

10. It may take a couple days of swirling the jugs now and then to get the sugar all dissolved. Then add water up to the neck.

11. After waiting one more day to make sure the mixture won't foam up out of the top, I put a masking tape label on each jug, noting batch number and the date it was mixed. Then I move the jugs off the kitchen table to a shelf (which happens to be in my bedroom, but could be anywhere), and I leave it undisturbed for many weeks (4 months is ideal).

12. When I start drinking the wine, I pour it from the same gallon jug it ferments in. A sediment develops at the bottom, so I stop pouring when I get down to the bottom inch or 2 and start using the next jug. When there's enough room in the newer jug, I marry the 2 by pouring the dregs that's left into the newer jug. After one day of settling, I can resume pouring from the newer jug. I wash out the empty jug using a bottle brush and re-use it when I mix the next batch.

13. The way to do it, so you don't have to wait 3 or 4 months while the wine is fermenting, is to get a system going like a pipeline. Mix wine periodically and add it to the right side of the shelf, while taking each oldest jug in turn from the left side. Keep moving the jugs over to the left as space opens up on the left side.

Variations: I've made wine using other fruit juices, but I've found that grape juice is really the best, also the cheapest. Above all, avoid cranberry juice, or any mixture containing cranberry. Cranberry appears to kill the yeast, and it absolutely will not ferment.

Wine can also be made from grapes or other fresh fruit. I make a small amount of wine from grapes each year, but I don't have a fruit press, so it's a much harder process that requires 3 separate filterings, thru a colander, thru a strainer, and finally thru a fine cloth. But the result is a richer, full-bodied wine.

DIY: Making Dandelion Wine

By Matte Resist

There are about as many recipes for dandelion wine as there are dandelions. They're all pretty similar, with the differences being mainly how you put the same ingredients together, how often you cook it, and strain it. I mixed a couple recipes together to come up with mine. I started with 2 quarts of tightly packed dandelion flowers. (Flowers and small leaves only, no stems) Many of the recipes would tell you to use a glass or a stone crock, but I didn't have one big enough. One recipe said I could use plastic, so I did. I used a very clean 5-gallon bucket with a tight fitting lid. (I found out that the main reason to use something besides plastic, is that it gives you a clearer wine. Mine is sort of cloudy, but it's mostly an aesthetic problem, not a taste one.) I put the dandelions in the bottom and poured one gallon of boiling water over them. The recipe I was using called for one thinly sliced orange and one thinly sliced lemon to be put in at the same time, but I didn't have one, so I did what another recipe said and added the fruit after the water was lukewarm (and after I had gone to the co-op and dumpstered an orange and bought a lemon).

After 5 days, the mixture should be strained through cheesecloth (you can usually buy it at the grocery store). Add 3 pounds of sugar and a packet of yeast, and let sit for another 3 days. Then strain the mixture again (through cheesecloth) and bottle. The bottles should be cleaned very well, sterilized with bleach and then rinsed very well. I used an old gallon jug, and a smaller bottle. Some recipes say to cork lightly, some say don't cap or cork. I think the worry is the bottles exploding. Probably the best way to prevent this is to have an airlock. I put an unlubricated condom onver the top of the bottle(unroll it first), and put a rubber band around it to hold it tight. This will allow the CO_2 to escape, but not allow oxygen in. When the condom starts to deflate, you can cap it. The wine should sit for 2-3 months at least. A number of the recipes said not to drink it until winter solstice. (As with any wine, if it tastes really nasty, don't drink it. Supposedly, bad wine will make you quite ill.)

I finally got to taste my first batch of dandelion wine. We broke it out on New Years eve and poured a small glass for the few people hanging around the house. The consensus seemed to be that the wine was good, but much stronger than normal wine. Nikolas said that it was more like a liqueur or dessert wine. If you know anything about making wine, you don't add sugar to make a wine sweet. Sugar is what the yeast feed on, which makes alcohol. Your standard homemade wine takes about 2 cups of sugar (2 1/2 if you like it a bit more stout) per gallon of juice. This recipe makes just over a gallon of wine, and uses 3 pounds of sugar!

I MADE MY OWN 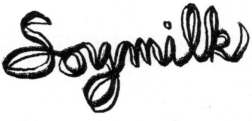Soymilk

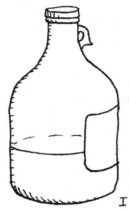

WHEN I WAS AT MY FRIEND STEVE'S HOUSE, HE HAD MADE HIS OWN SOY MILK & I THOUGHT "COOL! I WANT TO DO THAT TOO!" SO I DID. I GOT THE RECIPE FROM SOY NOT OI! IT WAS CHEAP & EASY. I SOAKED 2½ CUPS OF DRY SOYBEANS IN WATER OVERNIGHT. THE NEXT DAY I PUT 1 CUP OF THE SOYBEANS ALONG WITH 2½ CUPS OF WATER INTO THE BLENDER, BLENDED IT UP, PUT IT IN A BIG POT, & THEN REPEATED THIS UNTIL I HAD CHOPPED UP ALL THE BEANS. THEN I COOKED THEM ABOUT 20 MINUTES. NEXT I GOT AN OLD T-SHIRT TO USE AS A FILTER. I PLACED IT OVER A LARGE BOWL & POURED THE STUFF INTO IT. THE SOYMILK FILTERED THRU THE SHIRT INTO THE BOWL & THE BEAN PULP STAYED IN THE SHIRT. I FLAVORED IT WITH HONEY & VANILLA BUT NEXT TIME I WANT TO TRY COCOA OR NUTMEG OR CINAMMON. I USED THE BEAN PULP TO MAKE FAKE TUNA, & SOY BURGERS. YUM!

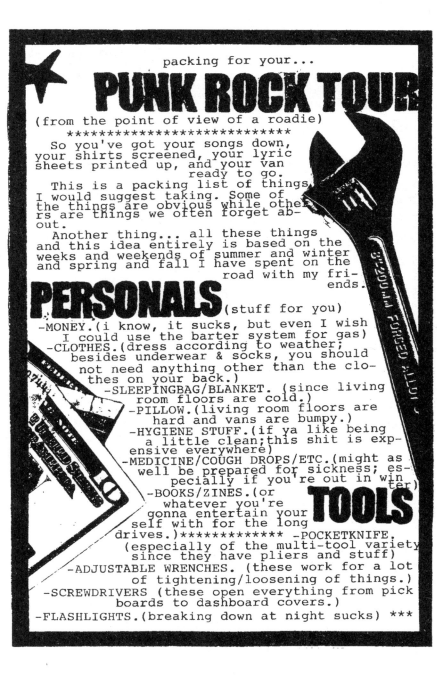

packing for your...

PUNK ROCK TOUR

(from the point of view of a roadie)
****
So you've got your songs down,
your shirts screened, your lyric
sheets printed up, and your van
ready to go.
This is a packing list of things
I would suggest taking. Some of
the things are obvious while othe
rs are things we often forget about.
Another thing... all these things
and this idea entirely is based on the
weeks and weekends of summer and winter
and spring and fall I have spent on the
road with my fri-
ends.

PERSONALS (stuff for you)

-MONEY.(i know, it sucks, but even I wish
I could use the barter system for gas)
-CLOTHES.(dress according to weather;
besides underwear & socks, you should
not need anything other than the clothes on your back.)
-SLEEPINGBAG/BLANKET. (since living
room floors are cold.)
-PILLOW.(living room floors are
hard and vans are bumpy.)
-HYGIENE STUFF.(if ya like being
a little clean;this shit is expensive everywhere)
-MEDICINE/COUGH DROPS/ETC.(might as
well be prepared for sickness; especially if you're out in winter)
-BOOKS/ZINES.(or
whatever you're
gonna entertain your
self with for the long
drives.)************* -POCKETKNIFE.

TOOLS

(especially of the multi-tool variety
since they have pliers and stuff)
-ADJUSTABLE WRENCHES. (these work for a lot
of tightening/loosening of things.)
-SCREWDRIVERS (these open everything from pick
boards to dashboard covers.)
-FLASHLIGHTS.(breaking down at night sucks) ***

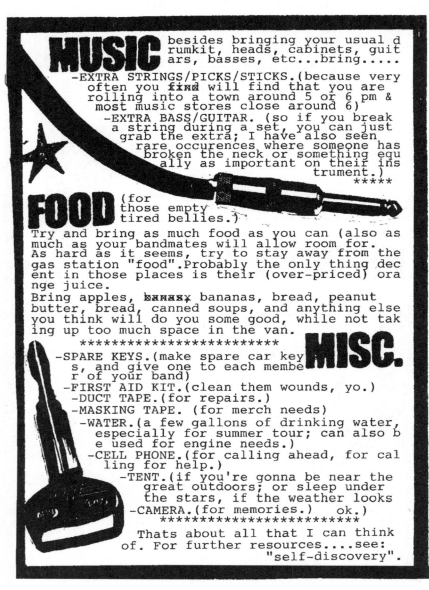

MUSIC

besides bringing your usual d rumkit, heads, cabinets, guit ars, basses, etc...bring.....

-EXTRA STRINGS/PICKS/STICKS.(because very often you find will find that you are rolling into a town around 5 or 6 pm & most music stores close around 6)

-EXTRA BASS/GUITAR. (so if you break a string during a set, you can just grab the extra; I have also seen rare occurences where someone has broken the neck or something equ ally as important on their ins trument.)
*****

FOOD

(for those empty tired bellies.)

Try and bring as much food as you can (also as much as your bandmates will allow room for. As hard as it seems, try to stay away from the gas station "food".Probably the only thing dec ent in those places is their (over-priced) ora nge juice.
Bring apples, banasy bananas, bread, peanut butter, bread, canned soups, and anything else you think will do you some good, while not tak ing up too much space in the van.

****

MISC.

-SPARE KEYS.(make spare car key s, and give one to each membe r of your band)

-FIRST AID KIT.(clean them wounds, yo.)

-DUCT TAPE.(for repairs.)

-MASKING TAPE. (for merch needs)

-WATER.(a few gallons of drinking water, especially for summer tour; can also b e used for engine needs.)

-CELL PHONE.(for calling ahead, for cal ling for help.)

-TENT.(if you're gonna be near the great outdoors; or sleep under the stars, if the weather looks

-CAMERA.(for memories.)   ok.)
****

Thats about all that I can think of. For further resources....see:
"self-discovery".

TIPS FOR STAYING FIT ON THE ROAD:

① WASH YOUR HANDS A lot.

② DON'T SHARE BOTTLES, Cigarettes, Cups, Joints, Forks, OR ANYTHING Else That could 'SPREAD' GERMS.

③ BRING YOUR OWN Pillow AND SLEEPING Bag. USE it All The tiME. EVEN iF SOMEONE Lets You USE ThEiR BEd, USE YOUR OWN BEdding ON top OF THEiRS.

④ DON'T GET WASTED. It BREAKS You down FAST.

⑤ BRING YOUR OWN MicRophONE

⑥ LAY OFF Excessive CAFFEINE. It BREAKS Down YOUR imMUNity

⑦ Eat vEgetables. They'Re CHEAP AND KEEp You up AND RockiN.

⑧ STAY AWAY FROM DiRty ToWELS. USE YOUR own towel.

9. EAT VITAMIN C, Echinachea + Multi vitamins.

10. DON'T BORROW OTHER PEOPLES' DIRTY CLOTHES.

11. GET SOME SLEEP.

* REMEMBER: EVERY NEW TOWN HAS A BRAND NEW SET OF GERMS JUST WAITING TO ATTACK. I don't get sick as much as i used to. I BREAK RULE 2 & 4 SOMETIMES AND IVE PAID THE PRICE. WATCH OUT FOR THESE DREADED COLD & FLU VIRUSES. They CAN REALLY RUIN A TOUR AND HURT YOUR SHOWS

P.S. WEAR a HAT. A Nice WARM Hat. WHEN it gets COOL

**Warning: this is all about Menstruation.
Squeamish folks proceed at your own risk.**

The first time I got my period, I didn't know what it was. A sticky brown paste in my eighth-grader briefs and an ache in my gut that felt like gas were not quite what the Judy Blume book and the school nurse's movie had prepared me for. I thought I'd somehow shit my pants without knowing. But when I returned to the bathroom to find the same stain in a second pair of undies, it dawned on me. I was utterly confused: periods were supposed to be red, not brown, and they certainly weren't supposed to show up until I'd gotten rid of my braces and grown big boobs. Really big boobs. Feeling betrayed and horrified, I stuffed maxipads stolen from my mom into the crotch of my cotton briefs and didn't tell anyone. I wore red shorts for a week and prayed that no one could hear the telltale *crispity-crisp* sound the pad made as I walked. By the time my next period arrived, as red and syrupy as I'd originally expected, I'd adjusted a little to the idea. I told my mom, and even mastered the fine feminine art of tampon insertion all on my own, a situation which altered my entire outlook on menstruation. While tampons didn't really change the fact that I considered my period something messy, painful, and embarrassing that I was going to have to live with for the next 35 years, they at least let me ignore it: I couldn't see 'em, couldn't feel 'em, and I certainly couldn't hear 'em. At night I braved all logic and slept with them in, during the day I kept a wad of them in the sack full of black eyeliner and hairspray (it was the eighties, okay?) that I lugged everywhere with me in high school, and the rest of the time I counted down the months until menopause.

Thirteen years and 156 periods later, I still can't bring myself to use a disposable maxipad (and I never did get big boobs), but otherwise my opinion of periods, and of tampons as the best remedy for them, has changed tremendously. At first I just started paying attention to how much waste the little buggers generated - around fifteen paper wrappers, applicators, tampons, strings, plus a box and instructions, per month - and switched to the bullet-shaped, no-applicator variety. These were more easily hidden in one's pocket, but they also required a more intimate relationship with one's anatomy. I gradually got over being grossed out and squeamish about it, and actually stopped ignoring my period and it's accompanying paraphernalia long enough to learn a thing or two about tampons.

MENSTRUAL CREATURES

FROM OUTER SPACE!

What I learned scared me. See, the tampons you buy at the drug store or in the feminine products aisle of the grocery are all bleached with chlorine to make them that lovely, "sanitary" snow-white color. One by-product of this chlorine bleaching process (which is also used for stuff like paper) is a lovely chemical in the organochloride family known as dioxin. Dioxin, for those of you not yet in the know, is one of the most carcinogenic substances on earth. It builds up in human tissue and cannot be eliminated by the body, so even small amounts can add up to eventually cause cancer. Chlorine-bleached tampons have been found to contain trace amounts of the chemical, and since tampons hang out three to seven days a month in the most absorbent area of a woman's body for 35 years or so, it's reasonable to assume that some of that nasty stuff will leak into you sooner or later. And even if it doesn't, the dioxin created in the bleaching process will eventually end up in the environment, where it becomes part of the food chain and does it's dirty deeds to the rest of the planet.

As if this weren't enough, I started to learn the real deal about toxic shock syndrome (no, not the band). From the innocuous little warnings included with every box of 'pons, I always had the impression that TSS was a freak thing, treatable with antibiotics, that might involve a trip the local hospital in really severe cases. I was wrong. TSS is caused by a fairly common bacteria (staphylococcus aureus, actually) which regularly vacations in a certain wet and warm area in around 15% of all female bodies. Generally it remains in a dormant state, much like retirees in Florida. But sometimes when conditions are right (especially when it get a little oxygen, food and a place to grow, all of which are supplied by most tampons), it decides to go crazy, Daytona Beach style. The bacteria itself is not necessarily harmful, but while it parties on, it pumps out a toxin that causes low blood pressure and damages organs and extremities. Even if antibiotics are administered (and currently there is only one or two antibiotics to which s. aureus is not already resistant), they don't eliminate the toxin, which must be filtered out slowly by the body. Although many women get mild cases of TSS and never know it, eventually building up resistance to the bacteria, the effects of severe cases include permanent organ damage, loss of fingers, toes and limbs (yes, they *fall off*), and death.

Fortunately for you, ladies, there are alternatives, and I've even taken it upon myself to play guinea pig in order to facilitate you making a well-informed decision about your choice of menstrual products. My first foray into the alternative menstrual product scene came in the form of all-cotton, non-chlorine bleached tampons. See, most of those major label 'pons (like Tampax, Playtex, etc.) are made with a blend of cotton and rayon fibers. Rayon has been shown to be a more hospitable breeding ground for s. aureus than cotton; hence, eliminate the rayon, and hopefully lower the risk (so far there have been no reported cases of full-blown TSS related to all-cotton tampons). These fellas are also completely biodegradable, and since they aren't bleached with chlorine, there's no dioxin to worry about, in you or the food chain. Another bonus is that these tampons are usually made by small, women-owned companies, rather than big icky corporations (punk rock). Having already grown accustomed to bullet-shaped, no-applicator style tampons, making the switch to all-cotton was no big deal for me, but if you're an applicator addict, it might take a couple tries. They were also a bit more expensive, and the string seemed to have a tendency to get more damp (it is, after all, cotton), but basically it was an easy transition for me to make, and I've used them for over three years.

My next experiment involved using the fabled sea sponge. These are the medium sized natural "sea silk" sponges found in art supply stores and cosmetics aisles, and I'd been hearing their praises as inexpensive and reusable (although not vegan) blood catchers for a few years. Before using it for the first time, I boiled mine for five minutes to sterilize it (as recommended by several different sources) and unfortunately watched it shrink in the process. I persevered, despite the suspicious chlorine smell emanating from the boiling water, running it under cool water, squeezing it dry, and stuffing it just inside my vag so that I could be sure to reach it later (some ladies tie or sew strings to them). While it was definitely the most comfy menstrual product I'd ever used, I was still worried about the chlorine smell, the fact that the sponge itself was harvested from waters around Taiwan (I called the company to check), and the knowledge that at least one case of TSS has been linked to sea sponges, so I aborted the experiment early. For anyone interested in attempting such a thing (at their own risk, of course), I recommend trying to find organic sponges (or those grown in the cleanest possible waters). My friend Rachel, a dedicated sea sponge user, suggests buying a good-sized sponge and cutting it down to size, and then microwaving it while damp instead of boiling it; she claims it won't shrink or get all chewy like mine did. She also cautions ladies to be sure they have a good grip on the sponge when removing it the first few

MENSTRUAL CREATURES

times, since blood-soaked sponges bear an uncanny resemblance to vaginal tissue. Don't forget to take it out and rinse it every few hours, soak it in vinegar and let it dry between periods, and get a new one if you use it when you've got any kind of vaginal infection so you don't get the ick again.

My experience with the <u>Keeper</u> was far more successful. The Keeper is a menstrual cup, so it collects menstrual blood instead of absorbing it, thus decreasing the risk of TSS. It's made of soft gum rubber by a small, woman-owned company, comes in two sizes and one lovely shade of reddish-brown, and can be used for up to ten years (very earth friendly). The Keeper's size was a little intimidating at first (it kinda looks a little like a miniature toilet plunger without the handle), but you fold it lengthwise to insert it, and can even use a little sex lube to make it easier. Once it's in, it pops open, and then you give it a little turn and maybe a soft tug to create a suction seal. I got a display sample from the company which had a hole drilled in it with a little chain attached (which I removed so I could see what it felt like), but even so it seemed to seal okay. I could kind of feel it at first: I felt sort of "springy" inside, which I assume came from the little bit of pressure it places on the vaginal muscles and surrounding organs. After a little while, I didn't notice it anymore. While I had a little leakage thanks to the hole, it was otherwise fine as long as I removed and emptied it whenever I used the bathroom. Removing it, though, can be a trick. There are tiny holes in the Keeper which are supposed to aid in releasing the suction, but I still don't quite have the knack, and usually ended up tugging hard and then spilling some of that lovely ruby red girl juice on my hand. If you're the sort of person who's bothered by that stuff, the Keeper probably isn't for you, but for everyone else, just practice at home a little and take a damp paper towel or two into the public restroom stall (or really shock 'em and rinse it in the sink... punk as fuck!).

The <u>Instead</u> menstrual cup is a little easier to use than the Keeper. Shaped like a cross between a jellyfish (without tentacles) and a little pink spaceship, Instead fits further up in the vagina, in the area near the cervix like a diaphragm. I was kinda pissed when I got it because it's packaged in lavender plastic and designed to be disposable (so annoying), but it ended up being so comfortable and easy to use that I grudgingly forgave them (plus, I am a woman with a plan). You just fold the cup in half lengthwise and slide it in past your pubic bone, and there it hangs out for up to twelve hours, although   you might want to check to make sure it's still in

FROM OUTER SPACE!

place after you use the bathroom. The cup holds a fair amount of fluid, so I noticed I felt a little "sloshy" sometimes, but that's not hard to get used to, especially since there's no dry, irritated tampon feeling. Like the Keeper, removing it can be a bit of an adventure, although there's no tug of war with your reproductive organs. It's just really important to pull the cup straight out when you're in a sitting position (not down, like a tampon); otherwise the back edge of the cup tips up, spilling blood, and more painfully, banging your cervix. I made this mistake once, and it hurt so bad I accidentally threw the cup across the bathroom, flinging blood from the toilet to the sink in a lovely arc... One cool thing about Instead is that you can have sex while wearing it, which is great if you're trying to practice safer sex (yes, HIV can be present in menstrual fluid) or if you have a squeamish partner who isn't down with earning his or her red wings. The cups' biggest drawback is their disposable design (the packaging warns vaguely of the risks of "vaginal infections"), but since they're pretty sturdy, I've taken to reusing mine for the past few months. Of course, I would *never* recommend that you save yourself some money and do this, or that you sterilize yours every morning with a bit of vinegar or diluted alcohol and let it dry before you use it.

    Finally, in the interest of thoroughness and my own health, I actually faced my worst fears and tried out some reusable, <u>cloth menstrual rags</u> for sleeping. It wasn't nearly as bad as I expected. They're available in awesome bright colors and patterns instead of boring and un-punk medical white, so I got one heavy-duty set in red as well as one light-duty set in plaid. Both sets snap or velcro around the crotch of your underwear; they seem to work better with dainties other than boxer shorts, but they still do a pretty good job of keeping my plaids plaid (instead of polka dot). Washing them isn't a big deal at all: I just rinse them out every morning in the sink with some cold water and shampoo, and let them dry all day, and at the end of my period I throw them in the laundry with my socks (what kind of woman cares if her menstrual rags are stained?). If you're really broke or super DIY, they're not hard to make from scraps like old towels and sheets. Although I can't say I've quite gotten past that nasty diaper feeling yet, I'll admit that the flannel fabric is actually starting to feel sort of comforting next to my skin. And at least they don't make any horrifying crunching noises when I walk.

MENSTRUAL CREATURES

FROM OUTER SPACE!

<u>stuff:</u>
- all-cotton/ non-chlorine bleached tampons: most health food stores and co-ops, or mail-ordered from Bio Business International, 78 Hallam, Toronto, Canada M6H 1W8 (416)539.8548 or from Natracare, 191 University Blvd, Ste. 219, Denver, CO 80206
- The Keeper: p.o. box 20023, Cinncinnati, OH 45220; 1.800.500.0077
- Instead: many pharmacies and stores; 1.800.INSTEAD
- cloth menstrual pads:
  > bloodsisters: 12 Ontario East, Montreal PQ, H2X 1G8 (awesome colors and patterns, even silkscreened for your menstrual enjoyment!!)
  > rag hag: c/o martinez, p.o. box 2087, Poughkeepsie, NY 12601 (DIY punk pads!!)
  > gladrags: p.o.box 12571, Portland, OR 97212

<u>info:</u>
- sea sponges: Medea Books, 3739 Balboa #189, S.? CA, 94121; (415)666.3332
- The Period Conspiracy: Chlam Media Press 2504 Ravencroft Ct., Virginia Beach, VA 23454; cooties@rocketmail.com; www.bluedesign.com/cooties/
- Bloodsisters (Canada): 15 Ontario East, Montreal Quebec, H2X 1G8
- Blood Sisters (US): 5115 Texas Dr., K-Zoo, MI 49009; bloodsisters_mi@hotmail.com; www.a/cor.concordia.ca/~qpirg
- The Museum of Menstruation online (seriously amazing, ladies!) www.mum.org
- for copies of lots of good info that i have about alternative menstrual products and the dangers of major label tampons, send me a few bucks. a nice letter wouldn't hurt either.

Disclaimer:
Upon doing further research, I would like to qualify my statements regarding dioxin as not being scientifically proven. I don't want any women who've used grocery store tampons for decades to freak out and think they'll get cancer. The bleaching process still sucks for the environment, though, and I do still only buy organic unbleached applicator-free tampons.

((MENSTRUAL MASSAGE))

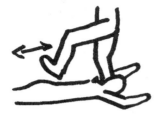

This massage is helpful in relieving cramps. Next time your partner is writhing in pain from cramps, give it a try. I've found that it doesn't completely get rid of cramps, but, while you're doing it, it feels good and helps relieve some of the pain.

Adapted from an anonymous untitled zine as well as my own personal experience.

How to do it:

The person with cramps should lay flat on their stomach. Be sure they tell you what feels good and what doesn't. It can take a bit of searching around to find the right spot, so be sure to communicate with each other until you find it. The person giving the massage should be barefoot and stand above the person with cramps. Stand with your feet on either side of their head, above their shoulders, facing towards their feet. You may want to grab a piece of furniture or stand near a wall so that you have something to grab onto to keep your balance. Keep one foot on the ground and use the heel of your other foot to hook into your partner's pelvic bone at the area where their lower back meets the top of their pelvic bone. Don't do it in the center of the back where the spine is, do it to either to the left or right of the spine. Begin a slow back and forth motion with your heel, applying pressure to the pelvic bone. Push the bone away from you, towards their feet. Try to create a rhythm where you push against the pelvic bone with your heel every $\frac{1}{2}$ second to a second or so. You and your partner's bodies both should start to rock in a rhythm with your foot thrusts. In order to work well, you may need to thrust more vigorously than you might imagine, and this position can get tiring after doing it for a little while, so be prepared. Occasionally, switch the foot you're working with, as well as the side of the pelvic bone you're working on.

HOW TO PEE STANDING UP

Adapted from an article by Marie in
Picking Up the Pieces #1

FOR LADIES

1) You probably want to try this in the shower first to get the hang of it so you don't piss down your legs and pants.

2) Make a V with 2 fingers and spread apart your inner lips of your vagina (labia minora).

3) Be sure to pull tight side to side and also pull upwards. This will angle your opening of your urethra (aka your pee hole). This is the tricky part, getting it angled just right so you don't piss yourself.

4) Pee as forcefully as you can. Start and stop the stream of pee as quickly as possible so it doesn't dribble all over you.

5) Play around a bit with how much pressure you apply with your fingers to get our aim down.

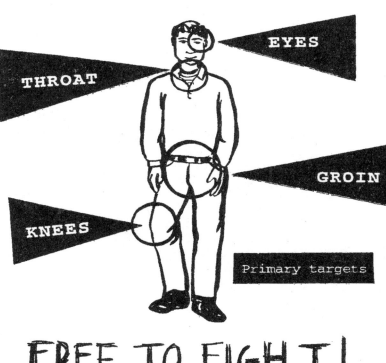

EYES

THROAT

GROIN

KNEES

Primary targets

FREE TO FIGHT!
an interactive self-defense project

Primary Targets

There are 4 primary targets on the body: eyes, throat, groin, and knees. Targets are considered primary because they have an involuntary or automatic response when hit. They are the most vulnerable. They are not pain dependent. All attackers, no matter how big and strong, have eyes, throat, groin and knees. Muscle and size can not protect the vulnerability of these targets. 25 pounds of pressure can bust out a knee and then an attacker can no longer chase us. Think about what happens when we get a piece of dust in our eye, imagine getting ten fingers in our eyes. And the throat, even gently pushing on our windpipe with our own hand makes us cough. When we hit hard and with multiple strikes we increase the likelihood of getting away safely. We use the strong parts of our bodies, such as our elbows, knees, hands/fists and feet against an attacker's weak parts, the primary targets. Remember it is the intention and internal will of the woman which are really important- if we choose to fight back physically commit 100% and hit with multiple strikes!

Female Sexual Play

(no penis required)

Adapted from an article in Girl Swirl #4, published by Taryn Hipp.

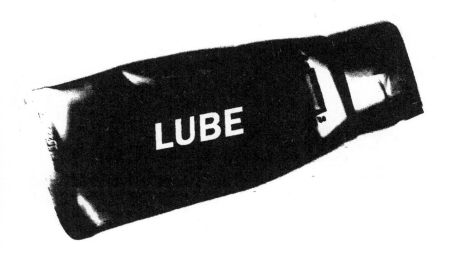

First thing's first – be aware of your fingernails. When it comes to sexual penetration, fingernails can be very uncomfortable, and can even cause damage. Ideally you want short, clipped nails that are smooth and round – no pokey or sharp nails! If you just have to have long nails, it would be a good idea to wear latex gloves to protect your partner. Of course, latex protection is also a good idea anyway to avoid any STDs or HIV. Some gloves are powdered and some aren't. It shouldn't really matter which you use, unless your partner is allergic to the powder (which is rare).

So, before you jump into any heavy activities as are described in this article, you need to first build up to them. Snuggling, kissing, touching, stroking, teasing and any other types of foreplay are essential. Build yourselves up by "getting in the mood" and slowly working your way to the point that actual penetration might be desired.

You'll want to have a bottle of water-based lube handy. KY and Astroglide are two popular brands. Don't use Vaseline or any petroleum based lubes. Smear plenty of the lube onto the hand you'll use for penetration. Before inserting, let the lube warm up to body temperature. A good trick is to place the bottle of lube in a bowl of warm water before you get started.

If and when you're ready for penetration, insert your first 2 fingers into the vagina. Move your fingers all around the vagina in a circular motion, keeping steady and firm pressure along the vagina walls as well as keeping a consistent rotational rhythm. Additionally, you can use your thumb to rub the clitoris while giving your inserted fingers a break. You can also occasionally, softly apply rhythmic pressure to the area just behind the pelvic bone, towards the belly. This directly stimulates the g-spot.

Meanwhile, you've got another hand just sitting there doing nothing. Here's a few things you can do with that other hand. Hold or rub your partner's body. Pinch or tease her nipples. Penetrate or gently massage the outside of the anus. Depending on your partner's comfort level and preferences they may or may not be interested in any of these. Communicate!

Of course, your mouth is also available for use too. You can do a variety of things with your mouth. Whisper hot, sweet, or sexy things to them. Play on sexual fantasies. Also, kissing, licking, and sucking other parts of their body, or even their clitoris, can be nice.

Women can have two kinds of orgasms – g-spot orgasms, and clitoral orgasms. It's possible to have multiple g-spot orgasms, and generally they increase in intensity as they progress. G-spot orgasms may not be easy to achieve initially if your partner has never had one before. It can take weeks or months to build up to one, and they can also be directly linked to the strength of her vaginal muscles.

If you and your partner are willing and able to take things even further, you may want to try vaginal fisting. This is an extremely intense experience, so be very sure that your partner definitely wants to try it before proceeding. Put your fingers and thumb together to form a shape like a duck bill. Slowly, with slight twisting motions, start to insert your fingers and thumb into the vagina. If you're able to get past your 3rd knuckles your hand will naturally want to curve into a fist inside the vagina. Again, doing this takes much time, trust, and communication.

Safer Sex is Better Sex

If you're going to be sexually active the number one thing you need to do to stay healthy is to use latex protection – condoms, gloves, etc. There's a huge range of types of condoms out there so it'd be best to experiment with different types to find what you like best. Some have Nonoxynol-9 which is a spermicide. This is good to avoid pregnancy, but gross for fellatio. Depending on what you're doing sexually, you may or may not want to get a kind with spermicide.

To put on a condom, pinch the tip, then unroll it onto your penis. Pinching the tip will help avoid an air bubble forming inside, which can lead to the condom breaking. For intercourse, use a water based lube. Not only does it feel better, but it also helps keep the condom from breaking. Whenever you withdraw the penis, be sure to hold onto the base of the condom to keep the penis from slipping out.

If a condom fails during intercourse remove it immediately. If pregnancy is a concern do not douche. Instead, insert a Nonoxynol-9 contraceptive foam and keep it in for about 15 minutes. You can call 1-888-NOT-2-LATE for information on emergency contraception. If STDs are a concern you can immediately urinate and wash your genitals with antibacterial soap. This is not going to be a huge help, but then, it can't hurt either.

During oral sex, herpes, and many other STDs can be transmitted from mouth to genitals and vice versa if protection isn't used. Again, condoms without Nonoxynol-9 can be used for fellatio, and either a dental dam or non-microwaveable plastic wrap can be used for cunnilingus or analingus. Be sure to apply lube to the receiving partner's side of the plastic wrap or dental dam.

After touching anyone's vagina, penis, or anus, be sure to wash your hands well with hot water and antibacterial soap before touching your eyes, mouth, or anyone else's genitals.

For any questions about STDs, HIV, or STD clinics in your area you can call the National STD Hotline at 1-800-227-8922. Above all, be safe, smart, and cautious. Be sure to educate yourself on all possible risks before doing something you're unsure about.

MALE SEXUALITY
Things They Never Taught You In Health Class (or On TV)

As a man, I feel cheated. As far back as I can remember, I have been forcefed nothing but lies about my sexuality. As a kid growing up in the Bible belt, sex was naughty. It was only for reproductive purposes between married adults and even then wasn't to be discussed outside the soap opera realm of gossip. In health class, they fed upon the pubescent fears of young men and instilled in us the idea that sex wasn't about pleasure or bonding or orgasms you can feel in your ears, but about a foot long penis and a submissive partner that would moan for a few minutes until you came. We are taught that the male orgasm is one and the same as ejaculation and that our most sexually potent parts are dirty and illegal in 17 states. Reinforcing these dictums are a million and one media images helping further define our sexualities into the anti-sensual, anti-pleasure traditions of Judeo-Christian culture.

Considering the overwhelming pervasiveness of this mental, emotional and sexual coercion, it is no wonder that so many men remain sexually unfulfilled (and shitty lovers to boot!).

Although an adequate dissolution of these bullshit constructs would fill several volumes and take years, here is a brief guide to help you on your way.

The Male Sex System Revealed
in Less Than Ten Sentences.

Let's say that you're getting sexually aroused. The three cylinders (cavernosi) within your penis (one surrounding the urethra that composes the glans or "head" and one on either side) expand, creating a hydraulic pressure in the arteries which feed them. The veins charged with the duty of releasing the blood for circulation back to the body's carburetor (the heart), responding to swelling of the penis, are cinched off and the erection solidifies. A few minutes or hours later, the tingly feeling around the swollen phallus becomes too much to bear and you succumb to your taunting organs. Two small glands below the prostate, called the cowper's glands, send a lubricating "grease" down the urethra, essentially paving the way for a friction free ejaculation. The testicles respond by contracting in towards the body, essentially "pushing" their bounty of sperm up through the vas deferens past the pubic bone and beyond the bladder. Soon thereafter, the sperm merge together with the creamy product of the Seminal Vesicle and then later with the watery harvest from the prostate gland (these latter two organs discharge a variety of substances in their respective packages; some that neutralize acids in the vagina, some that feed the sperm and some that inhibit the growth of bacteria). Less than three seconds later, the seminal cocktail comes flowing out into orifice, bedsheet or palms. Throughout this whole process lies the modest pubococcygeus muscle which, if properly empowered, can prevent, stop or otherwise manipulate this process by applying pressure to various points.

Ejaculation
Overseer of a Man's Sexuality.

First and foremost, ejaculation and orgasm are NOT the same thing. Although orgasm can and usually does appear immediately before ejaculation, the two entities are very different. Unfortunately, tenth grade health classes and mainstream media have convinced us that ejaculation and orgasm are one and the same, the culmination of all things sexual in men.

Ejaculation does tend to dominate male sexuality, as once the seminal soup goes flying, a coup de grace has been effectively delivered to the erection, and too often, a passionate night of lovemaking. As we know from personal experience and too many bad jokes on sitcoms, this event tends to occur far sooner than our partners would like and in most cases, deprives us of well deserved orgasms. By achieving an understanding of the mechanics behind ejaculation, we can learn to control it within ourselves and our partners and get on with more important things, like giving and receiving gasping, grasping orgasms that make your feet twitch.

Ejaculation is a biological response to particular stimuli. Just as a sneeze is a biological reaction to irritation in the sinuses or a fart the biological counterpart to mounting pressure on the nerves within the sphincter, ejaculation is the body's response to manipulation of the nerves surrounding the glans, head, and shaft of the penis. Once stimulation reaches its ejaculatory quota, the aforementioned process of seminal expungement starts. Here are some tricks that can help control ejaculation.

Piss before you start...
A build up of urine in the bladder places pressure on the prostate, seminal vessicle and pubococcygeus muscles within the male anatomy and helps exaggerate the urge to ejaculate. Similarly, just as an individual gets antsy when they have to pee really, really bad on a long car trip, so does a man get antsy when he has to pee during sex. Draining the bladder beforehand can help relax the entire experience and allow you to concentrate more on what you're doing.

Breathe a lot and relax.
Like when surfing, getting tattooed or anything else exciting, we often forget to breathe when we're fucking. Aside from generally speeding everything up, destroying our concentration and otherwise distracting us, the lack of oxygen actually stimulates the nerve clusters in our parts and helps that ejaculation work its way to the forefront of our mind. Furthermore, a lack of oxygen also tends to make people tense up, which again hinders the judicious execution of the sex act. So slow down there, hotrod!!! Take deeper breaths, relax, and start changing the rhythms, speed and directions of your thrusts...I guarantee your partner(s) will appreciate it.

Try a cock ring.
There are generally three different variations on the cock ring; one for the shaft, one for the testes/scrotum ("parachutes"), and those that do both. The basic purpose of a cockring is to help keep blood in your erect penis and/or to keep other fluids which may end your erection backed up in your parts where they belong. No need to go to that trendy bondage shop down the street to buy a brandname aluminum alloy cockring; you can make them yourself for a lot less. For the shaft type, go to the hardware store and try and find metal O rings that look about the same diameter (or a bit smaller) than your erect shaft. As a general rule, using a large diameter ring or plural rings is the most comfortable. Simply pull the ring around your shaft as you are getting near your point of maximum erection and make sure that the ring is tight, but not so tight your pee pee turns blue and shrivels up. You can also take that punky little leather bracelet with pyramid studs off your wrist and strap it around your shaft, just like it was designed for. When used correctly, shaft cockrings can give you some of the longest, hardest erections you have ever had.

The second kind, the parachute, fits around your scrotum and is designed to pull your testes away from your penis to fend off ejaculation. If you ever have felt your testes/perinial area during an ejaculation, you know that your testes pull up close to your shaft as ejaculation is occurring. For the parachute, one needs a ring or strap that can be pulled around the scrotum and over the testes into that nice little niche below the base of the penis. Oddly enough, that punky wristband you wear is possibly the right size to use for these purposes (indeed that is where the fashion came from in the first place!!!) and if you go to a sex shop and check out the selection, you will probably find that the designs are very similar. Just strap it on tight enough that it binds your balls below the strap and go to work. You will probably find that you will begin feeling parts of your body that you never knew existed before and that you can fuck for hours and hours without stopping. Of course, this does have some other effects on your bod. After a few hours of fucking without ejaculation, you may find that it feels like someone just kicked you in the groin or slugged you in the stomach. This is generally a good time to take it off and savor the surging ejaculation that often follows the removal of pressure. Sometimes after ejaculation is staved off for a spell, it is difficult to ejaculate for a little while without undue effort.

The third kind is a combination of the aforementioned shaft and parachute methods in which both a parachute and a shaft ring are worn simultaneously or a single ring used as both. Experiment and see what works best for you. (I have found that certain shower curtain rings, especially the big wooden ones, work exceptionally well for all purposes...they can be found at any DIY/hardware store)

The "push and pull method"

This uses many of the same principles as a cock ring, but without the equipment. As you feel the familiar tingling, surging sensation that signals the onset of ejaculation, reach behind you and pull your testes away from the base of your (or your partner's) penis. This will hold off the ejaculation and perhaps (at least in me) lead to the facilitation of a big fat, ear tingling orgasm.

Similarly, there is another trick that uses the same timing, but instead of grabbing your scrotum, take two fingers and push down on your perineum (the space between your testicles and anus). As you apply direct pressure to that space, you are actually pinching off the outersection of the prostate, vas deferens and the cowper's glands and ejaculation can be prevented, stopped, or at the very least, slowed. Furthermore, because of the prostate stimulation involved, this pinch can actually intensify orgasms tenfold. This trick, what the new agey Taoists call the "million dollar point," takes some practice to perfect, so don't get discouraged if it doesn't work the first few times.

The Glinch.

The Glinch is a neat little trick from a muscle you probably didn't know you had, the pubococcygeus. By flexing this muscle, you can also stop, prolong, or intensify an orgasm by pinching various parts of the ejaculatory cycle. To practice the glinch, drink lots of water or cheap beer, hit the john and start pissing. Once you get a good flow going, stop it. Then start again. Then stop. Then start. Stop. Start. Stop. Start. Each time you stop your flow of urine, you are helping build up this muscle surrounding part of your prostate, seminal vesicle and vas deferens. This muscle also contracts during orgasm and consequently, being buff from all your practice at the bar, can make your orgasm hit you in the ears. When you are feeling that spine chilling call from below, just squeeze your muscle and be amazed. The more you practice, the better it gets. This is also really handy for anal sex, because it gives you something to hold with.

The "Green Grass of Home".

If nothing else, just stop thinking about sex. Distract yourself from the tingling of your loins and the wonders of whatever orifice you are feeling on your nether regions. Some of my most profound political philosophy has arisen during the most heated moments of sex as I tried desperately to distract myself from the nagging pressure from below. Try turning your attention away from genitals (too much of sex is tied to genitals anyway) and try focusing it on nibbling your partner's ear or running your finger through their hair or caressing their back. Aside from distracting you and changing the mood of the sex a bit, it also feels nice.

Other Sex Stuff

Now that you have at least some idea of how to gain the upper hand on the seemingly omnipotent ejaculation leviathan, you can get on to exploring other things that can expand your sex life into areas you didn't know existed.

Go In the Backdoor.

I know full well that we've all been programmed into believing our rectums to be dirty places only enjoyed by perverts, but if this were what Nature intended, why are the most sexually sensitive points on the male body located within the rectal cavity? In fact, the composition of the tissues lining the "top" of the rectal cavity (bordering the prostate) are *exactly* the same tissues as those found on the top side of the vagina we've come to know and love as the "G-spot."

To casually stimulate the male "G-spot" inside the rectum, insert a clean, lubricated finger into the anus and gently massage the wall closest to the penis. About 1.5 inches to 2 inches up, you should find a nice spot that makes your head spin when touched. Try rubbing it while having sex or receiving oral sex and experience the best orgasm of your life.

As far as hygiene goes, simply wash your hands before and after stimulation, keep your nails trimmed and watch to not penetrate a mouth or vagina with an unwashed finger, lest you start a bacterial invasion.

Have Lots of Sex.

The best way to refine your sexuality is to have lots of sex. Period. Try multiple partners of both genders and experiment with neat and interesting positions. Follow your lust and find what makes you happiest and gives you the best orgasms. Masturbate regularly. Be open and communicative with your partners and ask them to do the same.

¡Never underestimate the power of a gasping, grasping orgasm to brighten your day!

DILDOS/BUTTPLUGS

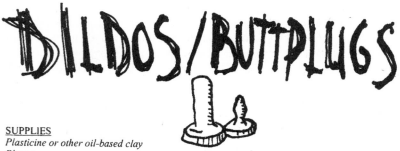

SUPPLIES

Plasticine or other oil-based clay
Plaster
Silicone, rubber, or Gelflex (make sure that whatever you use is "food safe," some silicones and rubbers have weird chemicals in them that you don't want to be putting in your body)

First you need to form the shape of whatever it is you want to make out of the Plasticine. This is exactly what your final product will look like so take your time, make it nice, smooth out any rough spots. You probably want to make it have a flared base to give yourself something to hold, and to avoid the whole thing accidentally slipping all the way in when in use.

Next, mix half of your plaster. There should be instructions about how to do this on the container. Pour the plaster into a shoe box that is just slightly larger than your dildo/buttplug. Once the plaster starts to firm up slightly, take your plasticine form and lay it down halfway into the plaster with the base butted up against the edge of the box. Then, in two or 3 spots around your form poke some small, shallow divots into the plaster with your finger. These will help later in locking your mold into the right spot. Let the plaster dry completely. Once dry, apply a layer of Vaseline to all exposed areas of the plaster. This Vaseline layer will help "release" the top layer of plaster, which you're about to pour next. Once the bottom layer is dry, mix the other half of your plaster and pour it into your container, filling it the rest of the way. Once fully dry, tear away the shoebox cardboard and peel your two halves of plaster mold apart.

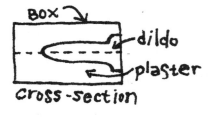

Pull out your plasticine form. You may want to put Vaseline on the plaster where your plasticine form was to help it release later on. Now, put your two plaster halves back together. Notice how the divots you made earlier help "lock" the two pieces together in the right spot. Now tie these two pieces together. Old bike inner tubes work really well for this purpose. You should have a hole in one end of your plaster mold where the base of the dildo/buttplug was. Pour your silicone/rubber/Gelflex into this hole. Do your best to avoid air bubbles. The best way to do this is to just put in a little at a time, then shake or knock the mold a bit to shake out any air bubbles. Keep doing this till you fill it completely. Let this dry for a few days.

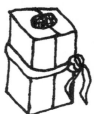

Once it's dry, pry open your plaster mold. Pop out your dildo/buttplug. You should be able to reuse this mold again and again to make more of the same form if you want. Now, have fun!

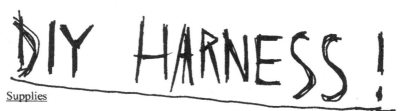

Supplies

Cockring
Velcro or plastic buckles or clasps
Sewing needle or sewing machine
String
Strips of fabric

Adapted from a homemade harness
diagram submitted for inclusion in the
HOw2 Zine, with a few alterations.

Here's how it works:

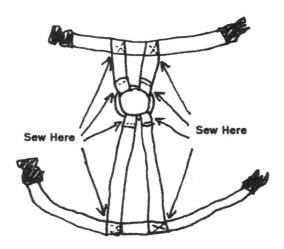

Sew Here   Sew Here

You can hold the different parts together with tape before you sew it to get the right
measurements. It's up to you what you want to use to hold the harness together when you
put it on. Velcro works ok, but may tend to come undone sometimes. Plastic buckles or
clasps (like from a backpack) tend to be better. So, stick your new homemade dildo into
the cock ring and go for it!

the rhythm method, STD's, Pregnancy scares, Late;

i had been reading about the rhythm method of birth
control when i was 19 ~~getting~~ in take back your life and
more thoroughly in our bodies, ourselves- a great resource
~~same~~ for women for many reasons, available at any library
or bookstore. i had just started dating a guy who lived
with me , we started using condoms each took hiv tests
and decided to try this. i got a basal thermometer at a
drug store and made charts every day to take my temperature

(a basal thermometer takes yer temperature to the tenth of a
degree. like 99.1, 99.2.. degrees farenheit, ya put it in yer mouth)

i also tried to be aware of changes in the elasticit of
my mucus (vagina!) - the tackier the less fertile and the
-ore elastic the more fertile, but i found it difficult
so metimes to tell. also the position of the cervix and
size of the hole and color change during your cycle,
but that is harder to tell on yer own.

i found out i have a 35 day cycle- very long & regular! it's only
day cycle- incredibly long and very regular. it only has
varied when i took a big bike trip where i got it for one
day each two weeks for two months.(a lot of excersize,
the food we eat and and our vices like drinking, or coffee
affects our body cycle.) so my ~~mmm~~ partner would remind
me to take my temperature every morning when i woke up at
the same time. we used condoms when i was ovulating- and
to be extra safe i would leave a 10 day period where we
didnt take chances without a condom. sperm lives 72 hour
in the body, but in case the period came early or late to
be safe id leave ~~six~~ 3-4 days before and after i thought
i was supposed to be fertile. your body temperature drops
~~xixmifixxxtix~~ during your period until ovulation and then
raises significantly for the rest of the month. but for
me, my temperature drops twice in a month.

everyones body is different. i ve had friends who will
never have a regular scheduled period, it can be 25-36 days
and they never know. travelling and changes in altitude
affect it too, it makes me crazy thinking about all the
factors that affect us. people who are transient, non-
monogamous, or have inconsistent period cycles should not use
the rhythm method.

this method is great for couples who are monogamous
willing participants and most of all DILLIGENT.
temperature must must must be taken everyday, hell
if both people take each others temperature it can
be fun . this is also good for women who are in
same sex couples to learn more about each others
bodies, or even for single women as a great way to
get in touch with yer body and not feel so naive
about it. it doesnt have to be about pregnancy
avoidance. it can be used to plan a child or for
self knowledge-empowering!

keeping charts was really empowering for me because i started knowing
what was really going on with me inside. i got a speculum and that was even better

my partner was good about learning with me, and he even
would remind me to take my temperature first thing when
i got up. he helped me take vinegar baths when i got a
recurrent yeast infection, and garlic clove inserts too.
unfortunately, what i didnt realize was that i had a real
bad yeast infection that wouldnt go away because i had
passed it to him and he'd pass it back to me and he was
never treated for one. so i had a bad yeast year.
we used this method for 9 months till we ended it.

Shared responsibility = shared learning= sucess = hot sex + fun,yo!

i kept track and kept using it with my next sexual relation
ship. but i was in lust, more insecure, too trusting and
even though id been tested for every std, he hadn't been.
he was constantly stoned and i felt weird asking him to be
responsible- he made mention to having probably left babies
all over the country. i found out he used to be a heroin
junkie. ~~xxxxxxxxxxxxxxxxxxxxx~~

~~xxxxxxxxxxxxxxxxxxxxxxxxxx~~ i started getting
freaked out, there were so many questions i never asked him,
so i went and got tested for every std again in case it
would be too late to see symptoms later.

sure, i was allergic to some condoms, but ive found ones
that im not allergic to. trojans SUCKED ASS. ive had the
blue and red ones pop (the only ones ive had break). my
favorites are lifestyles, and they are in the top 3 best
condoms in all clinical tests. when people say they arent
100% i have to say- they are like 98% effective, and the 2%
leeway is for people who dont pull out after ejaculation
and for people who roll the condom on bzza inside out and
still use it-even tho it's got precum on it. ~~~ if you
fuck up a condom get another! you can try unrolling it before you

put it on. you can get free condoms in most if not all cities
in New orleans at NOAIDS, drop in centers, planned parenthood,
Nowe Miasto, bars around town. for oral sex saran wrap!-
and hell, mint condoms or nonlubricated ones.
can be used or get flavored syrup from a sex shop or xx
make it yerself- just make sure there is NO OIL only water
based ingredients. oil rips holes in condoms. its good
to use the same precautions for the anus- hepatitis and
parasites and all sorts of stuff you can get from lickin
tare ass yo. i'm all for the revolution with latex! it can
be great fun, and hell, we learn our desires so lets learn
to love latex. its smooth, sheek, you can get all sorts
of colors. its like a wet suit. its also a way of minimizing
getting herpes or genital warts from partners that have
them (these are transmittable from the whole area yer
underwear covers). latex undies or liquid latex, making "it"
more than something that has to be quick!
ladies gotta be extra careful because allthexx stds xxxcan
creep into our cervix and cause cervical or uterine cancer.
the more we know, the sooner, the better.

ive only covered two types of birth control here becau
because they are the only two ive tried or would re-
commend.condoms are the most effective and reliable
of all devices. sponges, all those are crappy. the
diaphram is supposed to be really effective, but it can
also slip. must be put in hours before sex, so they are
no good for spontaneity. as far as the pill, deprovera
norplant, and ru486, ive heard horror stories of norplant
having to be removed for loss of feeling in the arm,
people getting pregnant any way, depression and mood
swings, and all sorts of things. as women, it is good
for us to bleed! it purges us of toxins and it is
cleansing. and these place all the responsibility on the
woman. fuck that! we all gotta be equally responsible
for this act which is xx a mutual experience. i say latex
is the way to go; condoms and dental dams. these protect
against stds. oral sex, anal sex, and vaginal sex are
all risky for hiv, syphillis,hepatitis b, warts,herpes,
gonorrhea. one last thing-the female condom- ive used
it and it feels like a plastic bag, its weird, it isnt
as effective as condoms,

some stds ~~and~~dont have symptoms, like chlamydia, or some
you may have symptoms for a couple days and they go away
and you never realize you   them until you stop
showing signs. some symptoms only show up when you have
unprotected sexual encounters with people also infected. so
i recommend being tested after every partner!we can be
a carrier or have a disease and not have symptoms or even
contract it ourselves. our health ingeneral being poor
will make us more susceptible or break out worse than
someone much healthier. just cause yer lover test negative
doesnt mean you will. parents without hiv can have babies
with hiv. for info on diseases, check our bodies
ourselves, ,the sexually transmitted diseases sourcebook,
or any other current text in the library.

Sex is fun, it shouldn't be scary, ignorance breeds fear,
knowledge lets us know what's safe or isn't. Have sex,
have fun, use latex yo!

EVERYTHING YOU NEVER WANTED TO KNOW ABOUT VAGINAL YEAST INFECTIONS*
*Until You Got One   by Julie Summers

Infuriating, exasperating, itching is the most common symptom of this,
the most common of vaginal infections, which accounts for nearly 20% of
outpatient gynecology visits. It is caused by a yeast-like fungus named
Candida, sometimes known as Monilia. (Yeast used in bread and beer making
is of a different kind, genus Saccharomyces, and is killed during baking
or pasteurization.)

C A U S E S
Up to 50% of normal women ordinarily have some Candida in their mouths,
digestive tracts, and vaginas. Why this usually harmless organism sometimes
causes trouble is not well understood. However, factors that increase
susceptibility are: pregnancy; diabetes; a high carbohydrate diet;
antibiotics; corticosteroids; birth control pills;   the last half of the
menstrual cycle; hypoparathyroidism; anything that lowers resistence, such
as smoking, fatigue, or travel; and possibly the use of commercial tampons.
During pregnancy the cells of the vagina store excess sugar which
feeds the Candida. A diet high in sugar or starch can have the same effect
in susceptible people, such as diabetics. (Some sugar in vaginal cells is
normal. It is released as old cells slough off, and is converted to lactic
acid by Doderlein's (lacto)bacilli which inhabit the vagina.)
Antibiotics kill beneficial microorganisms in the vagina, lessening
competition to Candida, thus permitting its rapid growth.

S Y M P T O M S
In addition to itching, the discharge of a woman with a Candida
infection may change to thick and curdy like cottage or cream cheese; it
is white in color; and does not smell bad. Some say it smells like dough
or baking bread, but that may be confusing since it is the way others
describe the odor of a healthy vagina. (The normal discharge is
non-irritating, clear to white or yellowish, and consists of Doderlein's
bacilli, sloughed-off cells from the vaginal walls, and some cervical mucus.
In addition to changing thruout the month it varies from woman to woman and
from one cycle to another in the same woman. For reference it is therefore
worthwhile monitoring a few cycles to become familiar with what is normal
for oneself. For a clear explaination of what to look for and how to record
it see A Cooperative Method of Natural Birth Control by Margaret Nofziger,
1976, 127 pages,   The Book Publishing Co., Summertown, TN 38483.)
P R E V E N T I O N
Attend to general health, including proper diet -- shun sugary foods.
(Manufacturers are required to list ingredients in decreasing order by
weight. However, they avoid listing sugar first, even when it is the heaviest
ingredient, by using different kinds. E.g., the following hypothetical
breakfast food is able to list wheat first, even tho it's 75% sugar! by
dividing the sugar among six different kinds:(2 oz.) wheat;(1 oz.) sucrose;
(1 oz.) maltose;(1 oz.) dextrose;(1 oz.) fructose;(1 oz.)lactose;(1 oz.) corn syrup.)
Don't douche routinely; it can upset the balance of a healthy vagina,
which keeps itself clean naturally.
On the other hand, the vulva (external female genitals) should be
washed, along with the rest of one's body, since stale secretions favor the
growth of microorganisms. Spread the lips and pull back the hood of the
clitoris so water can reach everywhere. To hasten restoring the skin's
normal protective acid mantle, rinse any soap (which is usually alkaline)
off well. (One women's health author recommends using no soap on one's
crotch, or limiting it to anus only.) Dry off well also since maintaining
dryness of the vulva is crucial in preventing Candida infections.
Avoid long, hot baths, which may encourage the growth of Candida.
Don't share towels. And wash your own often. If I use a towel more than

once between launderings I don't use it on my crotch, but use paper towels there instead. Do launder washcloths after each use, with very hot-water/bleach to kill any Candida.

Don't put anything into your vagina you wouldn't consider clean enough to put into your mouth. Wash sex toys such as dildos and vibrators with plenty of hot water and soap. In the event of recurrent infections, to help minimize   exposure to Candida, I would consider boiling or bleaching anything that was going to be placed in my vagina. (I'd boil it about five minutes; or soak a few hours in a solution of about 4/5 water to 1/5 household bleach. I'd be careful to rinse all bleach off well with plain water. Air dry, then store in a container treated the same way to be sure it's also free of Candida.) If a penis numbers among one's sex toys, I don't recommend boiling or bleaching (sighs from the men in the audience): soap and water will have to suffice. But condoms can be used, particularly if engaging in anal intercourse, in which case remove the condom immediately after the penis is withdrawn from the anus and before the penis may go on to touch the vulva or vagina. This is to avoid transferring Candida from anus or rectum to vulva or vagina.   and put on a fresh one

For the same reason, always wipe from front to back, i.e., from the vagina towards the anus: not visa versa.

Don't use "feminine hygiene" sprays, deodorant soaps, bubble bath, or scented toilet paper, which can all cause irritation or worse.

Around the crotch avoid tight or insulative garmets, or synthetics (e.g., stretch pants, pantyhose, or nylon panties) which trap heat and moisture, thus possibly stimulating growth of Candida. And wash panties, or other clothes that contact one's crotch, after a day's use.

Make sure your sexual partner (whether male or female) is clean and disease free. Although Candida is not usually sexually transmitted it can be. A condom affords some protection to a woman from an infected man and visa versa. (The infection in men is called balanitis. The penis may have visible lesions, or the Candida may be carried unseen under the foreskin or in the urine tube.) During oral-genital sex (homo or heterosexual) Candida of the genitals can be transmitted to the throat (where the infection is called thrush), or from throat to genitals.

Because injured membranes are more susceptible to disease, avoid painful or abrasive sexual penetration (whether with penis, fingers or dildo). If a lubricant is desired use a water based one, such as KY Jelly, not vaseline, which can clog vaginal pores, says Carol Berry, NP, writing in Medical Self-Care, 1980, Summit Books.

Because penetration (whether with penis, fingers, or dildo) can divide and spread the Candida colonies it may be best to abstain when infected, unless one notices no adverse effects.

T R E A T M E N T

Try abstaining from commercial tampons: for at least a number of months and see what happens. (For alternatives to commercial tampons -- in addition to pads -- see Everything You Must Know About Tampons by Nancy Friedman, 1981, 172 pages,   Berkley Books, 200 Madison Ave., NY 10016.)

If one suspects saliva as a mode of transmission: one may abstain from oral-genital sex for a while (and from using saliva as a lubricant during penetration) and see if doing so has any affect on one's infection. Also be attentive about where fingers touch, since they could possibly transfer Candida from one vagina to another, or from anus to vagina.

Theraputic douches: If the preventatives and above two measures don't eliminate one's Candida infection: before investing in a doctor, Nofziger says one can try douching with (white) vinegar: two tablespoons (4-5% acetic acid) per quart of warm water, once or twice a day for 5-10 days. The acidity is supposed to create an unfavorable environment for the Candida. If this fails one can try douching with buttermilk or yogurt (diluted to pass thru the douche tube) whose lactobacilli may repopulate a disturbed indigenous population, which normally keep Candida down, says Nofziger. (According to My Body, My Health, 1979, Wiley Medical Publications, no studies have been done on the effectiveness of internal or external use of yogurt for vaginal infections.) The douche bag should be only slightly elevated, so the stream isn't forceful. The yogurt must contain lactobacilli, but no sweetening, such as honey, fruit juice, sucrose, dextrose, etc. -- read the label.

Garlic: Another folk remedy is inserting a fresh clove of garlic into the vagina every 12 hours, for five days. Some recommend crushing the clove; others say not to. To facilitate removal gauze or thread may be affixed. (I have tried each of the above nature-cures with hopeful expectations but sorry to report, found them entirely ineffectual.)

Boric acid: The Contraceptive Technology Update of February, 1981 reported that researchers found boric acid treatment of Candida more effective than the much more costly prescription medication nystatin. The article said "Making your own size 0 gelatin capsules containing 600 mg of boric acid powder may cost only 31¢ for 14." The dose is one 600 mg capsule inserted vaginally daily for seven days followed by one capsule twice a week for three weeks. The article concluded "...preliminary observations suggest that a single weekly capsule of boric acid may prevent recurrent vulvovaginal candidiasis" (Candida infections). An article in Modern Medicine of February, 1982 discussing the same research stated that the researchers "have had no cases of acute or chronic toxicity after prescribing more than 2,000 courses [of treatment]." Note it's boric acid powder, not crystals; and that tampons can inhibit dissolution of the capsules.

Gentian violet: is effective, say Rein and Chapel, MD's, in Clinical Obstetrics and Gynecology, 1975, Harper and Row; and Frank and Frank, MD's, in The People's Handbook of Medical Care, 1972, Vintage Books. The drug nystatin is no more effective, say the Franks, but has found favor because it doesn't color everything blue, like gentian violet does.

To use gentian violet I painted my vulva with a 2% solution, and to reach the inside of my vagina I douched with ten drops of the 2% solution in one fourth cup of warm water. I repeated this once every second day, for a total of four applications, as the Franks recommend. My condition cleared up immediately. (Because gentian violet is a coal tar dye, and coal tars have been known to cause cancer in experimental animals, I queried the Centers for Disease Control (CDC). They were "...unaware of any studies linking the use of gentian violet to cancer or other serious conditions. However, long-term studies have not looked at the cancer risk in persons who have used gentian violet." Since gentian violet has long been and still is in use for treating thrush in babies, and is frequently used on animal sores, I feel there has been ample opportunity for acute adverse effects to have come to light. However, since cancers often occur decades after exposure, long-term effects seem uncertain. (And this may apply to other drugs as well.)

Nystatin (Mycostatin is one brand): The Contraceptive Technology Update article referred to above said "...seven to ten days after treatment 92% (45 of 49) of the patients treated with boric acid were cured...compared with 64% (35 of 55) of those treated with...nystatin."

In addition to vaginal suppositories, nystatin comes in pill form for oral administration. It is not absorbed thru the gut but is said to reduce intestinal Candida so the vagina is less likely to be reinfected from the anus. However, The Medical Letter's Handbook of Antimicrobial Therapy, 1982 (which references The British Journal of Venereal Disease, 55:36, 1979) refutes that idea, stating oral nystatin "has not been effective in reducing the relapse rate." Regarding toxicity, the CDC were "...unaware of any significant undesirable side effects of either nystatin or miconazole" (the latter being another prescription drug used to treat Candida).

Addendum: Vaginal yeast infections may be the body's way of saying no to unwanted sex when a woman is afraid to say it with her voice. Wise woman herbalist Susan Weed wrote this in her book on menopause and recommended practicing saying "NO!" Charlotte Kasl, in her book, If the Buddha Dated (et al) suggests regularly asking yourself what you want and how you feel. Set the chime in your watch and do it every hour. I discovered that what I wanted was to not have sex when I did it just to satisfy my partner (at least not often). Apparently I had some belief that it was my duty to satisfy my partner most of the times he wanted sex and that if I didn't, he would leave me. I became able to broach my feelings to my partner and now I am able to say no - with my voice - when I don't want sex, and my partner has accepted that without resentment. I have been free of yeast infections for some years now, but I'm not sure about cause and effect. Maybe aging has something to do with it, or might it be the fact that I very rarely eat refined sugar or flour or highly processed foods?

THE CURE FOR
BURNING HOT PISS
by Cat

This is the best way i know of to cure a urinary tract infection (UTI) or bladder infection.

• BASIC RECIPE •

½ oz. marshmallow root simmer in a covered pot with a quart of water for ½-1 hr. Take off heat. Then add 6 Tbs. Uva Ursi (or Manzanita) + 6 Tbs. dandelion leaf + a handful of horsetail plus a slice of ginger root. Let it sit for ½ hr. Drink it throughout the day and for 2 days after all symptoms are gone, if you don't want it to come right back.

simmering an herb in water is called a DECOCTION. Pouring hot water over a herb + letting it sit (steep) is called an INFUSION

UTI's are caused from bacteria (usually ecoli from intestines) getting to your urethra. Girls are especially prone to them because of the shortness in length of our urethras + the very close proximity of the opening to the ass, where lots of ecoli hang out. Sex is the most frequent infecting reason. It can be pretty awkward to talk about, but basically you have to make sure that anything that has touched the region around your ass, intentionally or unintentionally, does not get anywhere near your vaginal region. Unless it has been thoroughly washed inbetween. This means fingers, cocks, sex toys, anything. Sex isn't the only thing though. I got them a lot when i lived in a place with no water + couldn't wash myself or my clothes very often. Sometimes even just excessive amounts of caffeine can give you one if you've had one before. Some people just seem to get them for no reason. Being really dehydrated will do it too. ONCE YOU GET ONE, IT IS REALLY EASY TO GET ONE AGAIN, SO BE EXTRA CAREFUL

OTHER TIPS

- try to piss both before & after having sex

- wipe from front to back

- if you shit your pants, or a fart leaks out more than you expected, CHANGE

- drink lots of fluid (beer & coffee don't count)

- actually, beer & coffee are worse than not counting. Very much of either are bad when you have a UTI.

- don't hold your piss in-piss as often as you can. Don't give those bacteria any chance to adhere to the lining of your urethra. It's annoying, but you gotta flush them out.

It's important to start treating the infection as soon as you can. When you feel the first twinges & aren't even sure yet, start treating it. Drink tons of water. Drink cranberry juice. It does not need to be unsweetened. If the healthfood store where you can get herbs at is already closed, go get cranberry juice & drink a lot. It changes the pH of your urine which makes it inhospitable to the bacteria plus it makes the walls of your urethra more slippery so it's harder for the bacteria to stick to it. If you catch it soon enough, you can get rid of the infection with just cranberry juice.

* *
* IF YOUR LOWER BACK (= KIDNEYS) STARTS TO HURT A LOT OR IF YOU *
* GET A BAD FEVER, GO TO THE EMERGENCY ROOM. IT PROBABLY *
* MEANS YOU HAVE A KIDNEY INFECTION, WHICH CAN KILL *
* YOU OR FUCK YOU UP FOR LIFE. *
* *

THIS IS WHAT THE HERBS DO:

*if you can't find all the herbs in the
recipe, use the ones you can find, or
replace them with others that do the
same thing.

UVA URSI [arctostaphylos] - disinfects bladder + urethra. can be irritating
to stomach, so take with marshmallow. Don't use in pregnancy.

MARSHMALLOW [althea] - disinfectant + antinflammatory to urinary tract.
soothing to stomach lining

HORSETAIL [equisetum] - antinflammatory + astringent to bladder + urethra -
it takes tissue + shrinks it down.

DANDELION LEAF [taraxacum] - a strong, simple diuretic. That means it
makes you piss a lot. Also replaces electrolytes.

- other herbs -

PIPSISSEWA · good UT disinfectant (tincture 1-2 dropperfuls every 2 hr)
(can use instead of uva ursi)

JUNIPER · (berries for tea) tsp. crushed in cup of water. No in pregnancy
or if kidney problems or history of kidney problems. It's a
simple urinary tract disinfectant + it stimulates the kidneys.

CORN SILK · yes, the silk of an ear of corn. You can just eat it, "take
a dropperful 4x day of the fresh tincture. Diuretic + anti-
inflammatory to urinary tract.

other diuretics ... things to make you piss ...

NETTLES, CHICKWEED, CLEAVERS and there are many others.

How to Treat Head and Chest Congestion

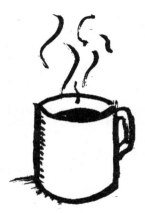

1. Find some dried hyssop (an herb). You may be able to find this at a natural foods store, a food co-op, from an herbalist, or possibly even in your own garden.

2. Add one teaspoon of hyssop to one cup of hot water and let it steep.

3. If you have head congestion, drink the tea hot. If you have coughs or chest congestion, drink the tea cool.

CONTROLLING HEMORRHOIDS NATURALLY
by Julie Summers

C A U S E S

Hemorrhoids, also called piles, are varicose (viz., puffed out) veins of the anal opening or rectum. They may be caused or aggravated by:

●Upright posture, which humans have evolved into while retaining anatomical features befitting quadrupeds, so unfortunately anal veins lack adequate support when one stands or sits.

●Pregnancy, in which case the growing fetus interferes with proper drainage of blood from the mother's rectal area.

●Straining when defecating, which pushes the hemorrhoids out.

●Foods that irritate the lining of the rectum, which according to The People's Handbook of Medical Care by Arthur and Stuart Frank, MD's (1972, Random House) fall into five catagories: seeds, strings, skins, stimulants (coffee, tea, alcohol), and spices. Highly irritating spices, says Nan Bronfen in Nutrition for A Better Life (1980, Capra), are pepper (black, white, and cayenne); cloves; ginger; horseradish; and mustard seed. Mildly irritating are allspice; anise; cinnamon; coriander; cumin; mace; and nutmeg. Chili and curry powders are combinations of spices, including irritating ones. Leafy herbs, such as oregano and basil tend to be non-irritating.

P R E V E N T I O N

Once one has hemorrhoidal veins, short of cutting them out, they're there to stay. Even if removed they may recur. Here are some things to do to avoid having these weak veins cause trouble:

●Exercise. Whereas sitting and standing-still allow blood to stagnate, movement tightens and relaxes the muscles, thus "milking" the blood back to the heart via the veins, which have one way valves at intervals along their lengths.

●Don't strain nor hold one's breath when defecating. To avoid the urge to force a bowel movement, eliminate constipation. In addition to regular exercise, which stimulates the intestines to empty, drink adequate water and eat plenty of fruits and vegtables, especially raw ones. Bronfen says "Carrots are one of the best foods to eat if you are afflicted with constipation. Eighty to 90% of their dry weight is fiber and it holds up to five times its weight in water". But she shows that wheat is even better: "It takes only about 2 ounces of whole wheat bread a day to double your stool weight".

Make sure the wheat is not ground too fine: "Dr. Peter Van Soest, a nutrition researcher at Cornell University, showed that although coarse bran and cellulose have a laxative effect, finely ground bran and wood cellulose...induce constipation..." reported Jane E. Brody in "Personal Health", NY Times, July 23, 1980. (Bran is an outer layer of wheat - removed from white flour - and although it may be purchased separately from the rest of the wheat I prefer it as it occurs in whole wheat, which I grind myself with a hand grinder.)

When defecating the posture that allows the muscles to work most efficiently is a squat, with knees drawn up to the chest, supporting the abdominal muscles. Tho U.S. toilets aren't designed for it, some foreigners accustomed to the squatting position reportedly assume one's feet are supposed to be placed on the seat. One North American puzzled long over footprints on her toilet seat until she discovered her foreign roommate didn't know anyone ever sat to defecate. The foreigner, in the mean while had pondered why the toilet was so high.

Most people probably won't want to perch with feet on the seat, but by elevating their feet with a stool they can simulate squatting and thus receive its benefits. At the end of a bowel movement twisting a few times to either side may encourage complete evacuation.

Although defecation shouldn't be rushed, don't spend more time on the toilet than necessary (e.g. reading) since it puts a strain on the anal veins. (A chair at least affords a continuous surface, unlike a toilet which leaves one's hemorrhoids literally out in midair.)

●Banish all suspect foods from one's diet for a few weeks or months then add them back one at a time and notice which, if any, cause distress. To do this you may have to read labels carefully since a spice like black pepper, for example, may be in anything from salami to mayonnaise.

I found that I can control my own hemorrhoid problem entirely by diet. I'm particularly vulnerable to whole sesame seeds (ground they don't seem to bother me). And when I eat apples, blackberries, or raspberries in quantity I have to be careful not to eat too many skins or seeds, which I do by peeling some of the apples and making juice from some of the berries.

T R E A T M E N T

If in spite of following the preventatives, your hemorrhoidal tissue flares up, here are some things that may soothe:

●Lying face down, or on the side reduces pressure in the affected blood vessels, and may ease the pain (note how the veins in the back of the hand shrink when the arm is raised, thus diminishing pressure).

●Fasting (ingesting nothing but water) or modified fasting (water and juices) may give relief by often minimizing the frequency and quantity defecated.

●If clots haven't formed, ice or astringents applied directly to the area may provide comfort, as I found before eliminating the problem thru diet.

●If clots have formed (palpable as hard lumps) the sitz bath, "which is nothing more than sitting in a warm tub frequently and for a long time, is probably the best thing you can do for swollen hemorrhoids" according to the Franks. The addition of corn starch (to the water or directly to the skin afterwards) may help alleviate itching. An alternative to baths is hot compresses for 15 minutes, four times a day.

●To avoid irritation when wiping, a bidet, or squeeze bottle or water as substitute may be gentler than rubbing. Pat dry. Robert Lawrence Holt in his book Hemorrhoids: The Problem, Personal Management, Medical Treatment (1977, California Health Publications, PO Box 963, Laguna Beach, CA 92652, about $8.50), recommends against using anything greasy (e.g. mineral oil) because it is not an effective cleanser and dirt tends to adhere to it. For further reading I recommend this book. It includes a discussion of cryosurgery (the rapid freezing of hemorrhoidal tissue) which is offered as a treatment when milder measures fail.

INKY'S DIY Lice Treatment
Ayun Halliday

1) Make sure you have lice. The easiest way to do this is to wake up scratching at your head as if you are being bedeviled by a great cloud of flies. If you have a child, you can distract her with an innocuous storybook in which none of the characters have lice, while you rummage around her scalp seeking the small brown bugs. If you find small brown bugs scampering purposefully amongst the stalks of hair, you may safely assume that you have lice.

2) If you have internet access, run a search engine on lice. You will find some amusing animated lice sure to make you feel exponentially itchier, as well as many advertisements encouraging you to purchase commercially prepared lice remedies. Most of these remedies have pyrethrum as their active ingredient. Pyrethrum is a deadly insecticide that you probably would not want to put on your head or the heads of your afflicted loved ones, particularly if they are under the age of 3. On the plus side, pyrethrum comes from a very pretty daisy that grows in Rwanda, and when you are travelling through a whole field of pyrethrum daisies on a foggy African morning, they give off a very pungent aroma that smells not at all unlike marijuana.

3) To prepare your own lice remedy, take about 2 cups of olive oil and add a few drops of rosemary oil, a few drops of lavender oil, and a few drops of tea tree oil. If your resources are low, skip the aromatherapy as its purpose is largely to make you feel pampered and healthy rather than bug-headed and skanky. The real aim is to smother the bugs in oil while greasing up their larvae for easy removal.

4) Massage the oil into your hair thoroughly and swaddle your head in a towel for at least an hour and a half.

5) Watch a video or listen to some cds and act as if you have the flu.

6) Dispatch a close friend to find a lice comb in a drugstore. The comb must have very fine teeth to remove the larvae which are smaller than grains of rice. Often a plastic baby's comb will have such fine teeth. Authorize your friend to buy several of these combs as the heavy oil in your hair will have them losing teeth like an old man eating jawbreakers.

7) Entrust this same friend with the very important job of combing through your hair. This is known as "nitpicking," so chose a friend with a reputation for being nitpicking in other aspects of her life as well. This friend should not be too squeamish. Wipe the remains of the bugs on a

paper towel. You can use a needle to pull their tiny crumpled corpses from the clogged teeth of the comb. Make sure your friend spends at least 45 minutes going over every inch of your head. Praise your friend lavishly. Every few minutes, inquire if your friend is remembering to get all of the larvae which look like little white specks, and can usually be found glued near the roots of your hair.

8) Shampoo and rinse your hair with a solution of 1/3 vinegar to 2/3 water.

9) Wash everything your licey head has touched, such as sheets and clothing, in very very hot water. For things that cannot be laundered, such as stuffed animals and feathered headdresses, put them all in a plastic bag and seal the plastic bag. Leave sealed for 2 weeks. Make sure not to share hats or pillowcases with family members, housemates, or friends.

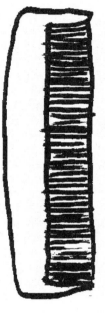

10) 1 week later, repeat steps 3 through 8. By this time any larvae your nitpicking friend missed in the original "comb and destroy" will have hatched.

11) Refrain from trying on "dress-up" hats in heavily trafficked public places. If your child attends elementary school, which is where many of us contract lice for the first and hopefully only time, you can smoosh a small amount of tea tree oil into your child's hair every morning before school as a prophylactic measure.

12) Rather than hanging your head in shame, be one of the first to come out of the lice closet by publishing a comic strip about your family adventure with lice. When your child is a teenager, you can drag the comic strip out to show all her friends.

DIY TOOTHPASTE

9 OUT OF 10 DENTISTS
PROBABLY WOULDN"T
RECOMMEND IT.

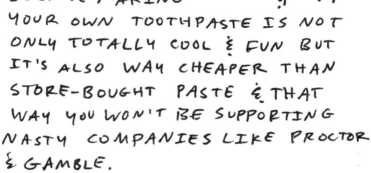

BUT WHO CARES?
BECAUSE MAKING
YOUR OWN TOOTHPASTE IS NOT
ONLY TOTALLY COOL & FUN BUT
IT'S ALSO WAY CHEAPER THAN
STORE-BOUGHT PASTE & THAT
WAY YOU WON'T BE SUPPORTING
NASTY COMPANIES LIKE PROCTOR
& GAMBLE.

AFTER A GOOD BIT OF RESEARCH &
EXPERIMENTATION THIS IS THE
RECIPE I'VE SETTLED ON - AT
LEAST FOR NOW:

2 TBS. CALCIUM CARBONATE - THIS
IS THE ABRASIVE THAT SCRAPES THE
GUNK OFF YOUR TEETH. IT'S BASIC-
ALLY JUST CHALK. I FOUND A
POTTERY SUPPLY STORE THAT SELLS
IT. ONE POUND COST ONLY $1.25!

HOWEVER, IF YOU FOR SOME REASON CAN'T FIND CALCIUM CARBONATE ANYWHERE YOU CAN TRY SUBSTITUTING CRUSHED UP TUMS OR ANY OTHER ANTACID PILL. I'D RECOMMEND GETTING THE UNFLAVORED KIND SINCE FLAVORED ONES USUALLY CONTAIN SUGAR & IT DOESN'T MAKE MUCH SENSE TO BRUSH YOUR TEETH WITH SUGAR!

<u>1</u> TBS BAKING <u>SODA</u> - THIS IS THE CLEANING AGENT. IT'S EASILY OBTAINABLE AT ANY GROCERY STORE FOR REAL CHEAP.

<u>1-2</u> tsp <u>GLYCERIN</u> - TO BE HONEST I'M NOT QUITE SURE WHAT PURPOSE THE GLYCERIN SERVES, BUT IT GIVES THE PASTE A CREAMY CONSISTENCY LIKE THE STORE-BOUGHT PASTES. IT MIGHT BE KIND OF HARD TO FIND. I MANAGED TO TRACK SOME DOWN AT A LOCALLY OWNED DRUG STORE. I THINK IT WAS LIKE $3.50 FOR AN 8 OZ. BOTTLE. NOTE THAT GLYCERIN IS NOT VEGAN, HOWEVER "VEGETABLE GLYCERIN" IS.

1/2 tsp PEPPERMINT EXTRACT— THIS IS TO GIVE YOUR PASTE A BIT OF FLAVOR SO YOUR PASTE DOESN'T JUST TASTE LIKE CHALKY BAKING SODA. IT SHOULD BE EASY TO FIND AT ANY GROCERY STORE FOR A COUPLE DOLLARS. YOU CAN ALSO TRY FENNEL OR CINNAMON OR ANYTHING ELSE.

A SMALL BIT OF WATER— THIS IS JUST TO MOISTEN YOUR PASTE A BIT, BE CAREFUL NOT TO PUT TOO MUCH OR YOUR PASTE WILL BE ALL RUNNY.

SO JUST MIX ALL THIS STUFF TOGETHER & GET TO BRUSHING. REMEMBER, FOR OPTIMAL DENTAL HEALTH BRUSH 3 TIMES A DAY FOR 2 1/2 MINUTES EACH TIME & FLOSS DAILY. FOR STORING YOUR PASTE YOU CAN CUT THE END OFF AN OLD TOOTHPASTE TUBE, SPOON YOUR PASTE IN, ROLL IT UP A BIT & STAPLE OR CLIP IT SOMEHOW.

FOLK REMEDIES

Many precious folk remedies and knowledge have been lost over the ages. In modern industrial capitalist societies we're taught to treat ourselves with weird medicines and chemicals that are not natural. Let's learn to heal ourselves in more natural and healthy (and cheaper) ways.

Some of these ideas are adapted from an article by Shyla Ann and Robnoxious in their zine Boy~Girl/Girl~Boy #2.

Garlic is great for boosting the immune system. If you feel a cold or other sickness coming on, or if you here of a "bug" going around, start eating plenty of it – 3 or 4 cloves a day if you can. Even if you're not feeling sick, it's still a good idea to regularly eat garlic, maybe just one a day during more healthy times. You need to ingest it raw to benefit from its super healing powers, but this can be kind of tough to do sometimes because garlic is pretty intense. A good way to ingest it is similar to the way you would take other medicine. First crush it up. Then get some water in your mouth. Then pop the garlic in and swallow it all down real fast.

Peppermint is good for soothing upset stomachs. After you eat all that raw garlic you may want to have some peppermint to soothe the burn. Also, peppermint is very easy to grow yourself. It takes off like a weed, so there's no excuse not to have some readily available.

Aloe is great for helping soothe and heal cuts and burns, including sunburns. It has Vitamin E in it. Just break off a piece and rub the gooey stuff on the inside of the plant onto your cut or burn.

Athlete's foot is caused by a fungus that grows on your feet. There's a really simple way to get rid of it, but people these days are so ridiculously scared of their own bodily secretions that some may not want to try this. I say "phooey" to that. All you have to do is pee on your feet. You may want to stand in a tub, or do it while you're showering. Just pee on your feet and let the slightly acidic ph of your pee work its magic. Eventually it should kill off that fungus.

Pests can be dealt with by using a number of different herbs. Cayenne sprinkled around doorways and windows will keep out ants and other bugs. Diatomaceous Earth can also be sprinkled will also kill many bugs in gardens and indoors without pesticides. Citronella, lavender, pennyroyal, and peppermint can all help in detracting fleas, ticks, and mosquitos.

Homemade Neti Pot
Trina

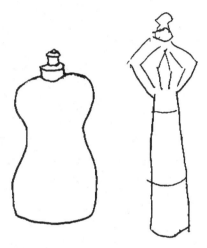

Neti pots are used in India to cleanse sinuses and for general purification. To make your own you can use a dishwashing soap bottle – the kind that looks like the Seattle Space Needle that you pull up to open. Make sure it's really clean, then punch a hole in it near the bottom. It works just like the fancy, store-bought ones. Fill it with warm water that has a touch of salt dissolved in it. Don't use too much salt or it will burn like hell. Tilt your head horizontally and put the bottle up the top nostril of your nose. Don't force the water. Due to the tilt of your head it will naturally be pulled through your nasal cavities and then drain out your bottom nostril. Be sure to do it on both sides. It will clean you right out!

HOW TO AVOID GETTING AN
EAR INFECTION

ACCORDING TO MY MOM AFTER GOING SWIMMING IN LAKES & RIVERS & PLACES LIKE THAT IT'S VERY EASY TO GET AN EAR INFECTION FROM BACTERIA IN THE WATER. THIS CAN BE EASILY PREVENTED THOUGH. WHENEVER YOU GET HOME FROM SWIMMING MIX UP A SOLUTION OF 50% VINEGAR AND 50% RUBBING ALCOHOL. GET SOMEONE TO POUR THIS INTO YOUR EAR & LET IT SIT FOR A MINUTE OR TWO. THEN TURN OVER & LET IT DRAIN OUT & FILL UP THE OTHER EAR. THE VINEGAR WILL KILL THE BACTERIA & THE ALCOHOL WILL HELP ANY WATER EVAPORATE OUT. MY MOM ALWAYS KEPT HER SOL- UTION IN A PLASTIC CON- TAINER LIKE THIS. I THINK THE SMALL NOZZLE MAKES IT EASIER TO AIM THE SOLUTION DIRECTLY INTO THE EAR HOLE.

D.I.Y. Pet Care Ideas

- To help your cat pass hairballs, dab some vaseline on its paws. The
cat will lick it off and it will go down and the hairballs will come up.

- For cats that are strictly kept indoors: plant some grass seed in a
clean litter pan or other wide, shallow container and keep it accesible
to your cat after the grass grows. Cats eat grass as a natural digestive
aid, and it may help deter the cat from chewing on any houseplants you -
have.

- Common plants that are toxic to cats: Azalea (Rhododendron), Laurel,
Dumbcane, Elephant's Ear, Mistletoe, Oleander, Philodendron,
True Ivy and Winter Cherry.

- Don't ever feed your cat or dog milk or lactose heavy foods, as they
don't have the proper enzymes to digest it. Milk can cause chronic
diarrhea in cats and dogs, and in the case of male cats, it can lead to
the formation of crystals in the urinary tract.

- Add fresh garlic (minced) or garlic powder to your pet's food to repel
fleas.

- If your cat is scratching up your furniture, rub any wooden pieces
with fresh Lemon Balm, or lay crushed sprigs of Lemon Balm on any
upholstered pieces.

Bonewits' Butt Rot:

A few years ago I was adopted by a stray cat that I called Bonewits.
After he lived with me for awhile, he suddenly got ill: no appetite,
very lethargic. After about two days of this, I discovered a wound right
under his tail next to his butt. It was awful! It looked like a very
deep, oozing hole about the size of a nickel. I was pretty scared for
him and also very broke, so I called up a vet to see if I could get the
cat in and work out some sort of payment plan. After I explained to the
vet what the problem was, he suggested I try putting saline solution
(contact lense cleaning stuff) on the wound for a few days. He said that
cats are prone to getting a certain bacteria in small cuts and scratches
that essentially eats away at the surrounding flesh. So I went down to
the grocery store and paid a dollar for some and started dousing what
had come to be known as "Bonewits' Butt Rot" with it. In a matter of a
few days it started clearing up and he got his appetite and energy back.
He continued to get similar wounds on various parts of his body on
occasion, but never as bad as the first. Whenever I saw a new one, I put
on plenty of the saline solution and they healed right up.

NON-TOXIC FLEACOLLARS

TO MAKE AN EASY NON-TOXIC FLEA/TICK COLLAR FOR YOUR DOG OR CAT
ALL YOU NEED IS :
- LONG STRIP OF MATERIAL 3" WIDE AND LONG ENOUGH TO FIT AROUND THEIR NECK AND BE TIED.
- THREAD + NEEDLE
- DRIED OR FRESH PENNYROYAL

1. TAKE THE MATERIAL, FOLD IT IN HALF AND SEW THE LENGTH OF IT — SO IT BECOMES LIKE A TUBE

FOLD   SEW   FINISHED TUBE

2. NOW STUFF IT WITH PENNYROYAL (YOU CAN ALSO USE SOME MINT THROWN IN, IF YOU WANT)

3. TIE IT AROUND YOUR DOG OR CATS NECK — LOOSE ENOUGH TO GET 2 FINGERS BETWEEN THE COLLAR AND THEIR NECK.

* YOU CAN ALSO USE A HANDFUL OF PENNYROYAL TO RUB ON YOUR FACE, ARMS, LEGS AND OTHER EXPOSED AREAS TO FEND OFF TICKS

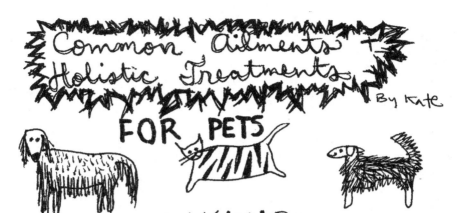

Common Ailments + Holistic Treatments
FOR PETS
By Kate

a L'il INTRO

So.... I grew up on a hippy farm. But while we ate vegetarian, organic, and fresh-cooked, cured our minor ailments with herbs and other "alternative" medicinals, our dogs, cats, chickens, rabbits, and goats pretty much got shafted. And this last summer when I worked on an "organic" farm, our goats there still were fed chemical-filled commercial crap. Our boss refused to give us time to make an organic food, let alone to give us the extra money it costs to feed organic.

Okay... so you don't have much cash. I know I sure as fuck don't. But I know a lot of lower-no income kids that are still pretty careful about what they put into their bodies. Well, the same types of crap that can hurt us can also hurt our pets. Cheap, crappy food is obviously bad for us, but since pet food has fewer regul-

LATIONS AS TO WHAT CAN GO INTO IT,
MANY FOODS HAVE INGREDIENTS WHICH CAN
BE DEADLY TO SOME ANIMALS. AND,
THE DISEASES THEY CAUSE; CANCER,
PANCREATITUS, KIDNEY AND LIVER PROBLEMS
; CAN COST FAR MORE THAN BUYING
OR MAKING A DECENT FOOD. THE SAME
GOES FOR MEDICINES. PRESCRIBED MEDICINES
THAT HAVE "SIDE EFFECTS" IN HUMANS,
DO THE SAME IN ANIMALS, SOMETIMES
ON A MUCH LARGER SCALE. (i.e.: ONE SIDE
EFFECT OF THE CANINE PAIN MEDICINE CARPROFIN
IS DEATH.) HERBAL, HOMEOPATHIC, AND VITA-
MIN THERAPIES ARE MUCH SAFER, AND
USUALLY MUCH CHEAPER AS WELL MANY
HERBS CAN BE HARVESTED IN YOUR NEIGH-
BORHOOD, HOMEOPATHIC REMEDIES ARE
CHEAP ON-LINE OR CAN BE EASILY STOLEN,
VITAMINS ARE OFTEN GIVEN OUT FREE
AT HEALTH CLINICS.
    THIS IS MOSTLY BASED ON DOG PROB-
LEMS, BUT MANY APPLY TO OTHER
ANIMALS. MOST OF THE DOSAGES ARE
A RANGE FROM CAT TO DOG. RABBITS WILL
BE ABOUT THE SAME AS A CAT, GOATS
AND VERY LARGE DOGS WILL NEED SLIGHTLY
MORE THAN THE HIGHEST DOSE, UNLESS
OTHERWISE NOTED. HOMEOPATHIC REMEDIES
ARE MORE CONFUSING AS TO THEIR ADMINISTRATION
SO YOU MAY WANT TO SPEAK WITH SOMEONE
WHO HAS USED THEM BEFORE, OR READ MORE
ABOUT IT. LOOK AT YOUR LIBRARY FOR A
BOOK CALLED DR. PITCAIRN'S COMPLETE GUIDE
TO NATURAL HEALTH FOR DOGS + CATS.

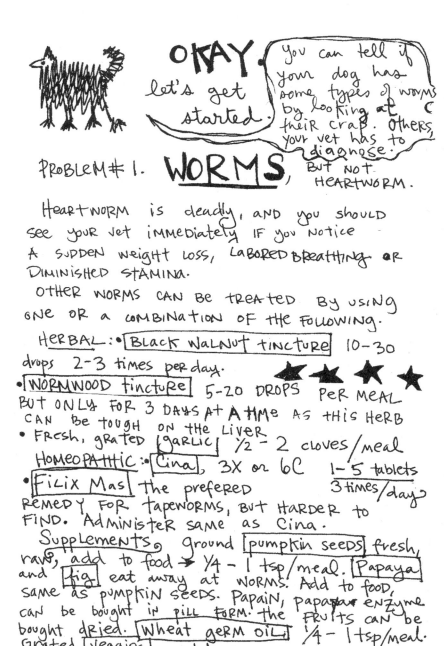

OKAY. let's get started.

You can tell if your dog has some types of worms by looking at their crap. Others, your vet has to diagnose.

PROBLEM #1. <u>WORMS</u>, BUT NOT HEARTWORM.

HEARTWORM is deadly, AND you SHOULD see your vet immediately IF you Notice A SUDDEN weight LOSS, LABORED BREATHING OR DIMINISHED STAMINA.

OTHER WORMS CAN BE TREATED BY USING ONE OR a COMBINATION OF THE FOLLOWING.

HERBAL: • BLACK WALNUT tincture 10-30 drops 2-3 times per day.

• WORMWOOD tincture 5-20 DROPS PER MEAL BUT ONLY FOR 3 DAYS AT A TIME AS THIS HERB CAN BE TOUGH ON THE LIVER

• FRESH, GRATED garlic ½ - 2 cloves/meal

HOMEOPATHIC: • Cina, 3X or 6C 1-5 tablets 3 times/day

• FILIX MAS the preferred REMEDY FOR tapeworms, BUT HARDER to FIND. Administer same as Cina.

Supplements: ground pumpkin seeds fresh, raw, add to food ➤ ¼ - 1 tsp/meal. Papaya and fig eat away at WORMS. Add to food, same as pumpkin seeds. Papain, papaya enzyme can be bought in pill form. the fruits can be bought dried. Wheat germ oil ¼ - 1 tsp/meal. Grated veggies, add to FOOD.

PROBLEM: 2: FLEAS

You can tell if your dog has fleas by looking at the dogs stomach, where fleas roam w/o the protection of fur on some dogs, or combing w/ a flea comb.

RINSE: 1 tbsp. [lemon juice] / 1c. water.

NUTRITIONAL: •1-2 tbsp. [nutritional yeast] added to each meal. Less for cats.
• 1/4 -1 clove fresh, grated [garlic] / meal.

HOMEOPATHIC: •[SULPHER] 30C. No food for 1 hr before + after administration. just give this treatment once. same for cats.
• You should wash all items which have come in contact with your dog. Add a good heaping of [BORAX] to each LOAD OF LAUNDRY.
• Sprinkle [BORAX] on your carpet, WHEN YOUR DOG WON'T BE ON IT, wait a couple hours, vacuum well, and bring your pup back in. You may have to do this a few times. [CRAP!] Yep, this totally sucks!

PROBLEM numero 3: CONSTIPATION
Is your dog straining to poop with no result? DON'T WORRY too much, if your dog has recently had DIARRHEA, this seeming-constipation is normal. DO WORRY IF your dog has been recently (±1 wk) SPAYED-straining can bust open the incision.

Step (1) add [vegetables] to pet's food. grated [garlic] is especially good. picky pets: put veggies in blender.

CONSTIPATION , cont.

step ②. IF, after a day or two, your mutt still has not taken a crap, keep adding veggies, but also add about 1 tsp of OIL (for a full size dog) to the meals. Olive oil is good, wheat germ oil is also good.

③ the OIL should do the trick, but if you are worried, or about 24-36 hours have gone by with nothin', try nux vomica 6C. This is a homeopathic remedy. No FOOD FOR 10 minutes before or after administration. give 1 tablet every 12 hours FOR up to 3 days.

④ So now you're probably pretty worried. Try giving a ¼ - ¾ tsp of vaseline (just once) to your pet. This should work in about 12 - 16 hrs. You should cover up important belongings wz your pet may have an accident. This is pretty tough on your pet, especially if you give them just a little too much.

⟵———————————⟶

• IF these things don't work, you should definitely see a vet.

PROB # 4 DIARRHEA

Both Diarrhea + constipation in pets are often signs of a larger problem. so you may want to take a stool sample into your vet regardless of whether they are cured or not.

• FASTING FOR 12 - 36 hrs is a good way to rid your pet's body of toxins that may be causing the diarrhea. Make sure your pet drinks PLENTY OF WATER, or SALT-FREE BROTH while afflicted, especially when fasting.

• DO NOT FEED TREATS, especially salty foods. You may be surprised to note the salt content of many treats. 1 tsp - 3 tablesp of kaopectate powder may be given up to every 4 hrs for 2 days as a cleanser / detoxifier.

• After the fast, a SLIPPERY ELM may be administered. Boil 1 tsp in one cup of water for 2-3 minutes. cats get ½ - 1 tsp, dogs 2tsp - 2tbsp, 4 times a day for as long as needed. It will help soothe your animals digestive tract.

• SMALL AMOUNTS OF PLAIN YOGURT may be given, to replenish good bacteria in the tract.

#5 MOTION SICKNESS

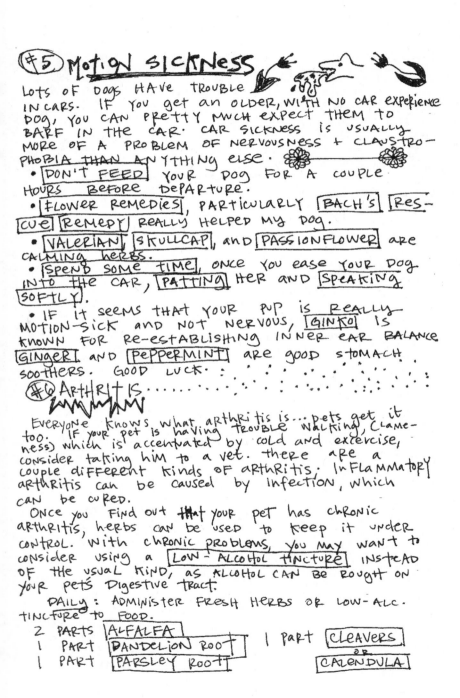

LOTS OF DOGS HAVE TROUBLE IN CARS. IF YOU GET AN OLDER, WITH NO CAR EXPERIENCE DOG, YOU CAN PRETTY MUCH EXPECT THEM TO BARF IN THE CAR. CAR SICKNESS IS USUALLY MORE OF A PROBLEM OF NERVOUSNESS + CLAUSTRO- PHOBIA THAN ANYTHING ELSE.

• DON'T FEED YOUR DOG FOR A COUPLE HOURS BEFORE DEPARTURE.

• FLOWER REMEDIES, PARTICULARLY BACH'S RES- CUE REMEDY REALLY HELPED MY DOG.

• VALERIAN, SKULLCAP, AND PASSIONFLOWER ARE CALMING HERBS.

• SPEND SOME TIME, ONCE YOU EASE YOUR DOG INTO THE CAR, PATTING HER AND SPEAKING SOFTLY.

• IF IT SEEMS THAT YOUR PUP IS REALLY MOTION-SICK AND NOT NERVOUS, GINKO IS KNOWN FOR RE-ESTABLISHING INNER EAR BALANCE GINGER AND PEPPERMINT ARE GOOD STOMACH SOOTHERS. GOOD LUCK.

#6 ARTHRITIS

EVERYONE KNOWS WHAT ARTHRITIS IS...PETS GET IT TOO. IF YOUR PET IS HAVING TROUBLE WALKING (LAME- NESS) WHICH IS ACCENTUATED BY COLD AND EXERCISE, CONSIDER TAKING HIM TO A VET. THERE ARE A COUPLE DIFFERENT KINDS OF ARTHRITIS. INFLAMMATORY ARTHRITIS CAN BE CAUSED BY INFECTION, WHICH CAN BE CURED.

ONCE YOU FIND OUT THAT YOUR PET HAS CHRONIC ARTHRITIS, HERBS CAN BE USED TO KEEP IT UNDER CONTROL. WITH CHRONIC PROBLEMS, YOU MAY WANT TO CONSIDER USING A LOW-ALCOHOL TINCTURE INSTEAD OF THE USUAL KIND, AS ALCOHOL CAN BE ROUGH ON YOUR PETS DIGESTIVE TRACT.

DAILY: ADMINISTER FRESH HERBS OR LOW-ALC. TINCTURE TO FOOD.

2 PARTS ALFALFA
1 PART DANDELION ROOT   1 PART CLEAVERS
1 PART PARSLEY ROOT   OR
                                                          CALENDULA

#6 arthritis, cont.

• FOR RELIEF OF especially bad ARTHRITIS, a
HOT COMPRESS IS ALWAYS NICE. IF YOU WANT,
YOU CAN MAKE IT INTO A POULTICE BY COOKING
DOWN WILLOW BARK → BUT NOT FOR CATS,
YARROW AND/OR COMFREY AND WRAPPING
IT UP INTO A CHEESECLOTH.

• WILLOW BARK (MAY BE SOLD AS WHITE WILLOW
BARK) CAN ALSO BE ADMINISTERED (TO DOGS
ONLY) IN PILL, TINCTURE, OR DECOCTION OR
TEA FORM (YOU CAN POUR IT OVER YOUR PET'S
FOOD). IT'S A GREAT ALL-NATURAL PAIN-
KILLER. (ALTHOUGH IT CONTAINS SALICYLIC ACID
(ASPIRIN) WHICH CAN BE DANGEROUS
TO CATS.

OTHER STUFF

• IF YOU ASK AROUND, YOU
CAN FIND YOURSELF A HOLIST-
IC OR HOMEOPATHIC VET WHO
CAN HELP YOU OUT WITH ALL
THIS.

• VITAMINS, PARTICULARLY A, C, AND E ARE
IMPORTANT TO YOUR DOGS HEALTH. IF YOU ARE
FEEDING A SUPERMARKET BRAND DOG FOOD,
YOUR PUP IS PROBABLY NOT GETTING ENOUGH.
EVEN IF YOU ARE FEEDING WELL, A SUPPLEMENT
CAN BOOST YOUR DOGS IMMUNE SYSTEM, HELP
FEND OFF DISEASES + DISORDERS, AND GIVE A
NICE, SHINY COAT.

• HERBS + OTHER NATURAL MEDS TAKE LONGER TO
WORK. FOR A CHRONIC PROBLEM, BE REAL PATIENT,
IT MAY BE A WEEK OR MORE BEFORE YOU NOTICE RESULTS.

new dog stuff

Ahh, a new home

• Depending on where you got your dog, it has probably been injected with all sorts of crap, i.e. vaccines. the same amounts of vaccine are given to a 2-lb chihuahua as to a 200 lb irish wolfhound. this, and the repetition of this, year after year, can add up to vaccinosis: where your pet actually gets diseases as a result of vaccines. you may want to try administering THUJA 30C - once a month (one tablet) for a few months after you get your mutt vaccinated, or possibly, not vaccinate her at all — you should talk to a homeopath or holistic vet about this one.

• Don't give your dog painkillers after sterilization surgery. this may make your dog think it can do things like jump up or race up stairs which can bust the gut on the incision.

• You may want to consider an anti-stress herb like valerian or a flower remedy, like the rescue remedy from Bachs.

Ahh... a new selection of things to barf on...

• good luck to ya.

...

The DIY Punk Rock Cat Diet
Mitch Freund and Michelle Downer

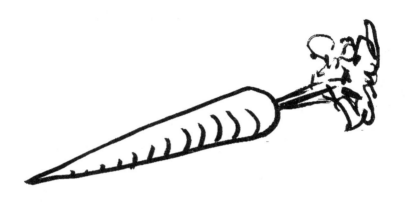

When we found out that the corporate mongers put cancerous growths and parts of meat unfit for human consumption into our kitty's diet we were disgusted. If it was unfit for us, why was it ok for our cats? We talked to our vet, read some books, and developed a recipe for cat food that supplies them with the best food you can find that also gives them all the nutrients they need. We developed it for our two 10 pound cats. Adjust amounts accordingly.

Per day, Per cat:
2 ounces meat (cooked for public health reasons) or steamed fish
2 ounces grain mix (see below)
½ teaspoon brewer's yeast
1/8 teaspoon bone meal or calcium gluconate powder

Preparing grain mix:
Buy grains in bulk. Use a variety of organic grains such as white or brown rice, oatmeal, buckwheat, millet, barley, cracked wheat, etc. Also use a variety of organic vegetables like broccoli, carrots, green beans, bell peppers, turnips, sweet potatoes, etc. Our cats love carrots, oatmeal, and sweet potatoes! You can make about a week's worth at a time.

Cooking grain mix:
This is for our two, 10 pound cats and lasts about a week. Adjust accordingly.
Boil ½ quart of water
Add 1 ½ cups chopped vegetables
Add 1 ½ cups grain
Reduce heat and simmer covered for 45 minutes
Dump mixture into a blender and mix until consistency of baby food
Keep refrigerated

Preparing the meat:
Cats should be fed cooked meat due to public health reasons. Feed a variety of naturally raised meats according to your cat's taste. Our cats like beef and turkey best. Pork or rabbit should be cooked well done. Cook meats with basil and garlic for taste and health benefits. Put it into a blender and chop it to a well ground consistency. At least once a week feed them organ meat like liver, heart, or kidney. One of our cats doesn't like liver very much and will only take a little at a time. You can cook about 2 – 3 days worth of meat, but keep it refrigerated.

When you have the meat cooked and the grain mix blended, measure off your serving, mash it together into a nice pudding, and feed your cat. There you go. Now your cat can eat "real" meat and you can flip off the corporate jerks.

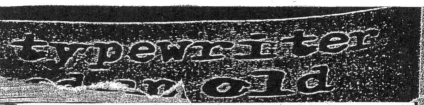

I get a lot of people writing me and asking about typewriter ribbons. Usually it's someone who has just purchased an old typewriter and is looking to get a ribbon for it, but doesn't know where to find one. Well, here is your first tip. If you buy an old typewriter, try to find one that already has a ribbon on it, or at least ribbon spools. Many typewriters use the exact same spools, but some use strange ones which you will have a difficult time finding. Often if you can't find them, your typewriter will be worthless. Also, if you aren't very familiar with typewriters, pay attention when you remove the ribbon so you know how to put it back in (assuming it was in right when you got it).

Once you have your typewriter, you may be able to buy the right ribbons from an office supply store. But what i prefer is to buy printer cartridges. You can often find them for really cheap, because nobody really wants them anymore. Look on the closeout/sale table. Try to find one that is either Nylon on Cotton (or silk, though i don't think they actually make those anymore) but not the tape type. Anyone that is 1/2" wide will be fine. Get the longest one you can find. I think 30 yards will fill up most spools. Then you just cut the ribbon, attach it to the spool and roll it on. Put it on your typewriter and write that earth shattering masterpiece that will put us all in our place.

matte resist

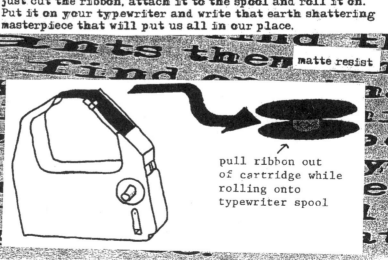

pull ribbon out
of cartridge while
rolling onto
typewriter spool

D.I.Y. BUTTONS

MY BAND MADE THESE BUTTONS WHEN WE WENT
ON TOUR. THEY'RE EASY TO MAKE, A GOOD ACTIVITY
TO PASS THE TIME DURING LONG DRIVES IN THE
VAN & ALMOST FREE! YOU NEED:

BOTTLE CAPS. THESE ARE ALL OVER THE
GROUND AND CAN ALSO BE COLLECTED IN
MASS QUANTITIES FROM ALL THE BEER
YOU DRINK EVERY NIGHT.

PULL TABS FROM CANS OF BEER. SAME
AS ABOVE — STRAIGHTEDGE BANDS CAN FIND
THEM LITTERING THE GROUND OR COLLECT THEM
FROM SODA CANS. THE REST OF US — DRINK LOTS
OF BEER.

SAFETY PINS. THIS IS THE ONE THING
YOU HAVE TO BUY. UNLESS THERE'S A
SAFETY PIN FACTORY IN YOUR TOWN. CHECK THE
DUMPSTER.

181 · Reduce, Reuse, Recycle

OK, SO THESE ARE REALLY EASY TO MAKE.
I DON'T KNOW IF IT'S JUST A REALLY CONVENIENT
COINCIDENCE, OR IF IT'S SOME SORT OF
CONSPIRACY BETWEEN THE BOTTLE CAP &
PULL TAB MANUFACTURERS, BUT IT JUST SO
HAPPENS THAT PULL TABS FIT
EXACTLY PERFECTLY INSIDE OF
BOTTLE CAPS. CHECK IT OUT! ⟶

FIRST TAKE A SAFETY PIN & HOOK
IT TO A PULL TAB LIKE THIS ⟶
THEN SET THE TAB DOWN INTO THE
BOTTLE CAP. GET A LEATHERMAN OR SOME
NEEDLE-NOSE PLIERS AND BEND THE EDGES
OF THE CAP OVER THE TAB TO CLAMP IT
IN. AND THERE YOU HAVE IT - A DIY BUTTON.
YOU CAN NOW PAINT THE FACE OF THE BUTTON
OR PUT STICKER PAPER ON IT OR WHATEVER
YOU WANT. PRETTY COOL, HUH?

HOT SAUCE SHAKER

LAST CHRISTMAS JENNY'S DAD MADE HOT SAUCE TO GIVE TO EVERYONE AS GIFTS. WHILE THE HOT SAUCE ITSELF WAS MOST EXCELLENT, I WAS ALSO JUST AS IMPRESSED WITH THE CONTAINERS HE PUT IT IN. HE USED THOSE LITTLE MINI BEER BOTTLES - SO SIMPLE, YET SO INGENIOUS. DRINK BEER, RECYCLE, & GET SOME DIY PUNK POINTS WHILE YOU'RE AT IT! THE BOTTLES WORK REALLY WELL BECAUSE YOU CAN SCREW THE CAP OFF & ON SO YOU CAN POUR THE HOT SAUCE IN THEN SCREW THE CAP BACK ON SO IT DOESN'T SPILL. ALSO, POKE A SMALL HOLE IN THE CAP WITH AN ICE PICK — THIS ALLOWS YOU TO SHAKE OUT THE HOT SAUCE IN SMALL SQUIRTS SO YOU DON'T ACCIDENTALLY POUR OUT TOO MUCH. AND IF YOU NEED TO SHAKE UP THE HOT SAUCE BEFORE YOU USE IT (IT SEPARATES AFTER SITTING AWHILE) JUST PUT YOUR THUMB OVER THE HOLE.

HOW TO MAKE A HANDY UTENSIL KEY CHAIN

I made this for myself a few months ago & it has been so great! There's a bunch of reasons why, & here's a few: 1. I always have a fork & spoon on me, so I'm always ready to eat 2. It saves water & dishes because I never have to wash tons & tons of utensils 3. A lot of times at pot-lucks or elsewhere the only utensil option is using crappy plastic forks & spoons that end up getting thrown away. But I always use my utensil key chain, so I don't have to contribute to this ridiculous wastefulness.

OK, so it's really easy to make this. Just get a fork & spoon. You might want to cut the handles a little shorter to make it more manageable. Drill a hole in the ends and then slip them on your key ring. VOILA! Now let's EAT!

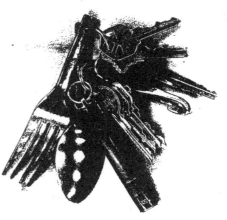

NOTE: YOU MIGHT GET A FEW FUNNY LOOKS USING THIS. I WHIPPED MINE OUT AT A FAMILY GATHERING ONCE & LATER MY MOM SAID ALL MY RELATIVES THOUGHT IT WAS WEIRD. OH WELL!

HOW TO TRAVEL-IFY YOUR BOOKBAG!

want to hit the road but hate those huge camping backpacks? got an old school backpack that's just dying to be put to better use? sick of carrying your sleeping bag in your hand, or tying it to your pack with ropes and letting it flop around?

HERE'S WHAT YOU'LL NEED:

★ your bookbag- duh!

★ your sleeping bag- ideally, you've got a mummy bag that scrunches up into a stuff sack. If you've got one of those heavy, pain-in-the-ass, flannel square bags, I guess this can still work - but I'll explain it assuming you've got the former.

★ one USED bicycle inner tube, ideally the thinner kind used in road bikes (as opposed to the wide, thick variety for mountain bikes.) You can find these in most bike shop dumpsters; or, if not, just go inside and ask for their old ones. if you find extra, save 'em! they're handy!

★ two sets of fasteners from the child safety belts in grocery store shopping carts. each set should look like this: ▭◖◗ ⊟▥ canvas belt these are also useful! (just cut 'em off of A → ← B carts in the parking lot)

★ waxed, preferably unflavored dental floss.

★ a needle - thinner is always better, but the eyelet should be big enough for the floss to go through.

★ scizzors.
that's it! let's get you started...

1. Cut the inner tube near the air nozzle; if there is any air in it, let it out, and don't inhale the white chemical dust that comes out. It will go from looking like this ⭕ to this ⌣. Lay it out as flat as possible.

2. Now position your sleeping bag up against the outside of your bookbag, like so:

SIDE VIEW   FRONT VIEW

the sleeping bag should be near the top of the bookbag; this distributes the weight much better. You are going to be making two straps, where the dotted lines are. they won't be adjustable but they will be a bit stretchy, as inner tubes are. they should hold the sleeping bag firmly, but not be too tight, so you need to figure out exactly how long they need to be. you may want to safety-pin the tops and bottoms of each length of inner tube in place and test it out.

wait, I'm getting ahead of myself! Just start out like this — much easier:
with sleeping bag in place (firmly held there!), align a length of inner tube running down the top of the backpack, from where the arm straps start to where the zipper is, and then down the sleeping bag about halfway. this will be the top portion of the left or the right strap. you should make the other top portion at the same time, so cut this length and then cut another piece of the same length.

3. On one end of each of these new pieces of tube, attach one of those shopping cart belt pieces - either use both "A" pieces or both "B" pieces. Stick the tube

2

through the space on each piece where the canvas belt once was; loop it around on the other side for a good inch or so, and sew firmly with floss. I make mine look like this: —that is, I sew an entire square on that inch that's looped around, so that it's extra sturdy.

Now once you've done that, you're ready to sew the other end of each of those pieces of tube to the top of your bookbag! There's a good 6 inches or so of space on the top of most bookbags, between the main zipper and the arm straps. Sew the straps along at least 4" of this, for good support. From the top, it should look like this: and the two straps should be about 8" apart for good balance. your new straps are firmly in place!

4. The best way to figure out exactly how long the straps should be is to just go ahead and sew the other cart belt pieces— let's say they're "B" pieces — onto two remaining, equally long pieces of tube (which should end up being much longer than you'll need; just halve whatever portion of tube is left at this point, making sure to cut off the air nozzle). Sew these on the same way you sewed the "A" pieces on. You'll end up with two of these: (except the straps will be longer).

5. Now clip those things you just sewed into the things that are hanging from the top of your pack.

Clipped together, these almost-done straps should dangle down nicely. So fit your sleeping bag back where you'd fit it before, now with these straps running over it. All that's left for you to do is:

pull each strap down tightly — but not too tight! — until it reaches your backpack again. It should be made to touch your backpack right at the bottom of your sleeping bag — not too high or low. That is,

right here!   not here...   or here, cus get it? good, my drawings suck.

That's the best way to keep it in place.
So once you've found that sweet spot to sew it all together at, you're set! Just like with the top straps, distribute the weight by sewing the strap down to your backpack for a few inches, like this:

—sewed down
(bottom of bag)

It might be tough finding a good place to sew it to on the bottom of your bag — oftentimes there are confusing pockets there that will get in your way. But you can figure something out. Happy traveling!

★ Cut up and manipulated in various ways, inner tubes can be used for lots of things! I sewed a long, narrow, vertical pocket on the side of my backpack to put my recorder in. You could do the same for a harmonica, stickers, toothpaste... ★!

MAKE A QUILL PEN

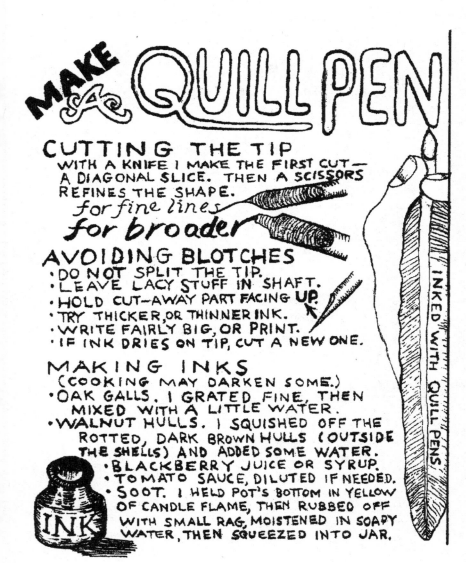

CUTTING THE TIP
WITH A KNIFE I MAKE THE FIRST CUT —
A DIAGONAL SLICE. THEN A SCISSORS
REFINES THE SHAPE.

for fine lines

for broader

AVOIDING BLOTCHES
- DO NOT SPLIT THE TIP.
- LEAVE LACY STUFF IN SHAFT.
- HOLD CUT-AWAY PART FACING UP.
- TRY THICKER, OR THINNER INK.
- WRITE FAIRLY BIG, OR PRINT.
- IF INK DRIES ON TIP, CUT A NEW ONE.

MAKING INKS
(COOKING MAY DARKEN SOME.)
- OAK GALLS. I GRATED FINE, THEN
  MIXED WITH A LITTLE WATER.
- WALNUT HULLS. I SQUISHED OFF THE
  ROTTED, DARK BROWN HULLS (OUTSIDE
  THE SHELLS) AND ADDED SOME WATER.
  - BLACKBERRY JUICE OR SYRUP.
  - TOMATO SAUCE, DILUTED IF NEEDED.
  - SOOT. I HELD POT'S BOTTOM IN YELLOW
    OF CANDLE FLAME, THEN RUBBED OFF
    WITH SMALL RAG, MOISTENED IN SOAPY
    WATER, THEN SQUEEZED INTO JAR.

INKED WITH QUILL PENS

INK

Everybody has something they want to keep private, but today's fast-paced e-world has made privacy fleeting and hard to find. I say, fight back against this creeping intrusion by building little pockets of privacy where you alone know the content!

How to make a Valuable Stash-Safe out of an 8-Track Cassette

Take the enigmatic 8-Track tape. Who hasn't admired its ugly resilience? The next time you're in a thrift store, don't pass the 8-Track by! Simply follow the instructions below and you too can transform this aloof art object into a stylish safety deposit box. Silly, subversive, and pleasurably hands-on, this Safe blends unnoticed into even the smallest 8-Track collection, making it virtually invisible to overweening parents, mooching roommates, curious siblings, snoops, fuzz, and other uninvited guests. Put that beguiling 70's aesthetic to work *for you and for your privacy!* It's fun, it's easy, and it's very, very practical.

Step 1
CHOOSING AN 8-TRACK
·Once shunned by hipsters and music buffs, 8-Tracks are now enjoying a renaissance, finding their way into exclusive music collections everywhere. This new-found "collectibility" can make locating just the right 8-Track for your Safe an adventurous pursuit.

Your first step is to rummage through the music bins at local thrift stores. Look for a tape that has three openings in its front, as shown in *diagram 1*. Both halves of the tape, as well as the label, should be securely intact. To all outside appearances, the tape should look ordinary and unaltered.

Step 2
TAKING AN 8-TRACK APART
Once you've located a suitable tape, your next goal is to separate it into halves.

To separate *this particular type** of 8-Track tape into halves, first locate the bonding sites *on the front of the tape.* These are the three little holes, as illustrated in *diagram 1*, where the two halves of the cassette are fused together. A small plastic nub should be visible inside each hole.

Using a thin, flat-blade screwdriver, push the nub in the top hole *toward the center of the tape* while gently pulling apart the two halves. *See diagram 3.* With a little finesse, the top part of the tape should separate into two pieces. Use the same procedure to unhook the locks in the lower right and left-hand corners of the tape. Remember to push the nubs *toward the center of the tape* while you gently pull apart each corner. *Note:* This procedure requires some mechanical skill to master, so I recommend that you buy a half dozen or so of these "snap-

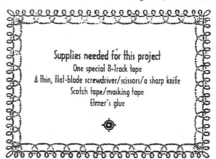

Supplies needed for this project
One special 8-Track tape
A thin, flat-blade screwdriver/scissors/a sharp knife
Scotch tape/masking tape
Elmer's glue

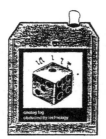

outside front

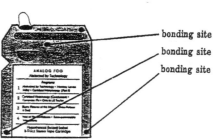

outside back

bonding site
bonding site
bonding site

Diagram 1

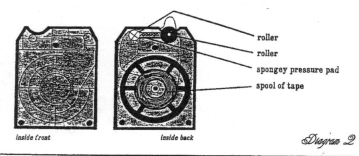

roller
roller
spongey pressure pad
spool of tape

inside front   *inside back*

Diagram 2

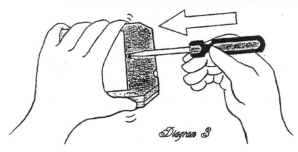

Diagram 3

lock" cassettes to give yourself tapes to practice on.
Besides adding a fashionable accent to your home's interior
design, a stack of tapes will also camouflage your Safe
more effectively.

Step 3
INSIDE AN 8-TRACK TAPE

Once you've separated your cassette into halves, remove
the spool of tape, the spongey pressure pad (Some tapes
come with pads mounted on metal prongs. Remove these, if
present.) and all extraneous plastic. Set everything aside.
The insides of an 8-Track tape are illustrated in *diagram
2.*

Note the storage space. To maximize your storage
potential, carve away all protruding plastic from the
center of the cassette using a sharp *knife*. Leave the
plastic at the top of the tape intact. Use masking tape to
cover any jagged edges.

Next, glue the rollers back into place, (*see diagram 4*),
and encircle them with a small loop of tape, (*diagram 5*).
This tape loop preserves the super-realistic look of your 8-
Track cassette. When your Safe is finished, the tape will
still look ready to play!

Tip for 8-Track enthusiasts: If one of your buddies
innocently picks up your Safe with the intention of playing
it, simply inform your friend that the spongey pressure
strip is missing from the tape, making it unplayable.

Step 4
PUTTING YOUR SAFE BACK TOGETHER

To close your Safe, simply align the two halves of the tape
and press them together until they snap into place. Be
careful not to pinch the tape loop in the seam between the
cassette's halves.

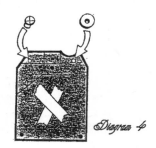

Diagram 4

*Use Scotch tape to splice the two
ends of the cassette tape together.*

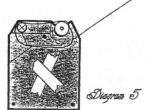

Diagram 5

* There is an astonishing variety in the designs of 8-Track tapes, and many styles
have hidden locking mechanisms that can only be properly disengaged with a 3/16"
drill bit. To preserve the appearance of your Safe, avoid tapes that use locking
mechanisms other than removeable screws or the "snap locks" described in Step 2.

Urban Foraging

An essential skill that should be acquired by all good little DIYers is the ability to scavenge for what is needed – to sharpen our senses and become aware of how and where we can find things without forking over the blood money. We can regain the ability to forage and utilize things that are often discarded or ignored. The beasts of mass production are dulling our power to create our own reality and to sustain both ourselves and our families/tribes. Of course combating this plague of corporate dominance over resources on the large scale may seem far out of reach, but for us urban dwelling folk, the solution may be lying right around the street corner in that big green "waste receptacle." They call it a dumpster – I call it a cornucopia.

There are other forms of urban foraging that are worth considering and exploring although they are often more subversive and less legal (think construction sites, back doors, lock-picks, sneakiness, and scams galore. Just don't be an asshole and don't get caught). However, I'm going to solely focus on the art of searching through trash, commonly called "dumpster diving."

First of all, we've got to get over the taboo of reusing people's trash. We have to learn to deal with the traumatizing experiences of elementary school classmates that chanted "trash picker" as you accidentally dropped your pencil in the garbage and dug to retrieve it. Those jerks are still out there yelling, complaining, and pitying you. I say fuck 'em! But if you've got the patience to talk to them I guess it's not a bad idea. You may want to tell them how most dumpsters aren't that gross or how seldom you see any roaches, rats, syringes, or dismembered body parts (although I've seen a few scavenger cats scare the shit out of people). Just be sure to finish the conversation expressing your disgust in the waste and overconsumption of our nation, then throw in a nice fact or statistic such as, "46 billion pounds of food goes to waste a year in the US," according to, um… those Food Not Bombs flyers which may not be a credible source to your average yuppie.

Anyway, the most obvious need to keep your body moving and your brain pumping at creative survival skills and good DIY ideas is FOOD. Learning to fuel ourselves without a degrading wage job should be one of the first things on all of our active minds. Until you can grow all your own food, successful dumpster scores are not only going to fill your personal quest for nourishment, but also will enable you to share your finds with everyone you know for days! So where to start? Get a VEHICLE (trucks and vans are nice, but a bike cart will also do). Map out your route and prepare for a sleepless night. Hit any big produce stands, grocery stores, donut shops, bakeries, bagel shops, or various food distribution centers (for example, most large cities have Frito-Lay centers) – check the phonebook. Compactors are the most common complication. I guess they came out of the brilliant idea that smushing trash makes it go away.

DESTROY these things without mercy. Dumpsters are also often locked, but there are several methods of circumventing this on a traditional dumpster. Try taking off the lid from the back or bending the rubber lid. For more difficult situations a snip from good bolt-cutters may do the job. Just be sure to have good etiquette and clean up after yourself. Maybe they'll think they forgot to put a lock on in the first place. Remember: think covert. You don't want to ruin it for other divers. If there aren't any other alternatives you may also want to simply try the front door. Ask for donations of expired/damaged goods. I suppose that doesn't have to be a last resort. It just seems much less fun.

Another important resource for DIY-minded individuals or groups is building materials. For general construction type stuff, poke around in the big industrial sized dumpsters located at demolition/construction sites in strip-malls or residential neighborhoods. Another place to score is often behind bicycle shops where spare parts are sometimes tossed. You can find rims, tires, chains, hardware, seats, tubes (which are useful for a variety of things), baskets, helmets, etc. Large, usable pieces of carpet scraps can be found at many carpet outlets. Furniture stores may have old or damaged chairs and furniture. Remember that all things can be either used with a little repair or salvaged for wood and hardware.

What about turning trash into cash (or credit)? This is very doable, but I'll keep it short. One option is scrapping metal: aluminum siding and doors, appliances with metal tubing. Also, items thrown away may be returnable for cash or credit, enabling you to purchase the necessary things you can't acquire otherwise. Places such as K-Mart are often a plethora of goods.

With your newly recovered scavenger mindset you will see things in a new light, as more than objects or products. All things that exist are made up of structure, simple or complex, and breaking down that seemingly useless broken exercise bike might create a foundation for your homemade cider press (in fact, there's a hell of a lot you can do by harnessing pedal power). How about broken computer hard drives? Before you smash it to pieces for the pure pleasure of it, try to pull out the super strong magnet – it could be useful. Once you adopt a forager lifestyle you will look at things differently. People often claim that dumpster diving is too dependent on industrial capitalism's waste to be glorified, but there is no refuting that it adds a perspective that is beneficial, if not necessary, in learning skills that will make us more independent and self-sufficient. If we are to create sustainable, healthy relationships with the planet and with each other, we need to change the way we view the resources available to us.

And one last quick point: don't blow money on shit you can get free.

11 places to dumpster dive

1. Bakeries-Bagel Shops-Donut shops(Krispy kreme mmm...) So many bread products you won't know what to do with it all, well I'll give you some hints, share it with your friends and soup kitchens offer it to random people on the street set up free bread stands harass people downtown to give you money for your products and if they refuse, beat them within an inch of their life or just call them funny names .

2. Grocery Stores- These fools throw away so much food it should be a crime. I don't know why grocery stores have a problem with shoplifters if they're just gonna throw it all away anyway. They throw away a wide variety of fruit and vegetables, pudding, cakes, eggs, bread, meat (I think that part will always be beyond my ability to ingest but if you have a carnivorous pet, they'll rip into that shit and its a lot better for the earth and its inhabitants than supporting dog and cat food companies) all kinds of food and a very high percentage is perfectly good (except of course that the food at corporate stores is genetically engineered and pesticide ridden and dairy just isn't good for you in the first place, but hey it's just as good as if you purchased it). Just use common sense in determining if it's not good and don't forget to wash it off, and don't forget to share. Lot's of stuff is still in it's package, natural and synthetic.

3. Bookstores and libraries- Sad but true. And ironically enough, many copies of fahrenheit 451 and 1984 have been salvaged from corporate bastards and public libraries. Please go salvage these fucker's waste. It's really sad to think of all these books never being read. Go!

4. Discount Stores- Big lots and the like throw away some fun stuff and I often wonder what's in the Toys R Us dumpster. Only a pair of bolt cutters will solve that mystery.

5. Whole Sale Florists- They throw away tons of flowers. And what better way to show your friends that you care about them than breaking in their house when their not there and putting rose petals all over their floor and filling their house full of flowers.

6. Plant Nurseries- they throw out live plants and dirt all the time. The plants just need some tender love and care. There is just something inherently evil about throwing away live plants, they'll get theirs in hell.

7. Drug Stores- We've scored hundreds of envelopes, tons of plastic Easter eggs, candy, just all kinds of random shit.

8. Pizza places- mmmm.... pizza

9. Ultimately , everything in our society is produced for consumers (a couple of exceptions). And, sooner or later this stuff is thrown away. So go to your neighbors house and jump on in. Apartment complexes are really good as well.

10. Colleges- At the end of the semester all of the students go insane and decide to throw away everything they own. It's really strange. But hey just more proof that college doesn't really make people any smarter (at least not in any area that counts).   a few college kids don't go insane but they are the exception to the rule.

11. Thrift Stores throw out some of the most fun junk. Go get it

Lot s of stores have compactors, and although these hideous machines are pure evil, the staff of WDTDD does not recommend that you take bolt cutters to their hydraulic lines. Nor does the staff endorse putting super glue in any locks of compactors that require keys to operate. Even though you would be doing a great thing by damaging these horrible machines, we request that you restrain yourselves from such awful acts of violence.

POLITICS OF PISS
Basic Graywater

It's pretty ridiculous that we use fresh, pure water to flush our toilets, especially when water, like all natural resources, is in a serious state of depletion. Pretty ridiculous that the water we use in the bathroom sink, that could easily be routed to fill the toilet tank, just drains away. Rivers are re-routed and dammed, valleys are flooded, all so that we can flush our toilets with sparkling water and have lush green golf courses in the middle of the desert.

Here's a couple of really basic things you can do to reduce usage.

There's a lot we can do, even in an urban environment and with little or no plumbing skills. This doesn't have to be some back-to-the-land homesteading style.

1. Disconnect the pipe under your bathroom sink so that it drains into a bucket. When it is 1/3 to 1/2 full (you'll soon figure out how much you need), it can be used to flush the toilet by simply pouring the water into the toilet bowl. It flushes by gravity, just like the normal flushing process; all the water pouring in pushes everything down the sewage pipe.

2. Keep a jug or bricks in the toilet tank, to reduce the amount of water that is used when you do flush the toilet.

3. Piss outside, or in the shower. Piss is good for plants that need extra nitrogen. (corn, for example)

4. Wash clothes in the shower. For watering the garden, you can use buckets or barrels to catch rainwater from the roof.

More advanced stuff includes graywater from your shower to water the garden, or an outdoor graywater shower; a pedal-power washing machine that also waters the garden; a fully composting toilet. For more information, get the GUERILLA GRAYWATER GIRLS GUIDE TO WATER for $3 + 2 STAMPS P.O. BOX 3831, OAKLAND, CA 94609

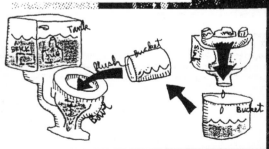

GUERRILLA SHIT COMPOSTING

→ SHIT: YOU SHOULD KNOW ←

So, we dumpster most of the food we eat, shoplift what we can't, monoculture coffee shops can't seem to keep their windows from getting smashed, and we just emailed the White House 1.7 gazillion times about the Jefferson Nat'l Forest 700 acre timber sale. We live, eat, and breath non-participation in a system we don't agree with. And yet, we still contribute to the most polluting, most land-stripping, most generally destructive "service" Capitalism has to offer: The Sewer System – we still shit in flush toilets, and we still flush it away. The system is shit, and we shit in it!

The sewer system is not only incredibly expensive to operate and maintain (yes, every time you buy a pack of smokes, you're paying for it!), it also demands an insane amount of energy and dumps millions of gallons of highly toxic chemicals into the environment and into our drinking water.

Let's get boring and take a look at some of the facts:

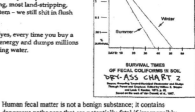

SURVIVAL TIMES
OF FECAL COLIFORMS IN SOIL
DRY-ASS CHART 2

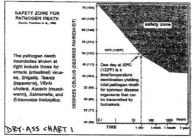

DRY-ASS CHART 1

The pathogen death boundaries shown at right include those for enteric (intestinal) viruses, *Shigella, Taenia* (tapeworm), *Vibrio cholera, Ascaris* (roundworm), *Salmonella,* and *Entamoeba histolytica.*

- Human fecal matter is not a benign substance; it contains dangerous pathogens that are potentially fatal if irresponsibly managed.
- Irresponsible management has led to plagues, typhoid, the Stock Market and more
- Hookworms, pinworms, and roundworms scare everybody, but:
- Hookworms: infect about 500 million
- Pinworms: infect 208.8 million – is not transmitted through feces
- Roundworm: infect 900 million – 1 million in the U.S.
- Pathogenic worms rarely, if ever, survive the composting process.
- Pathogens in general cannot survive outside their host for very long at all. In this case, the host is your up yer ass (see dry-ass charts 1 and 2)

- Urine does not contain ammonia! Ammonia is toxic while urine is sterile. Urine is very nitrogen rich. Nitrogen evolves into ammonia quite rapidly when it mixes with the air. Nitrogen is a valuable resource while ammonia is not. The nasty-ass "piss" smell is indicative of nitrogen loss, making it twice as evil.
- Don't turn your compost pile! For fuck's sake! Every time you turn it you lose a ton of nutrients. If, for instance, you turn it once every two weeks, you lose 75% of your nitrogen! Instead, use two compost piles and rotate them; fill one up, switch to the other. A backyard compost pile will not and has never exploded. Fuck urban legends.
- 5 billion gallons of purified water get flushed every day. In the U.S., groundwater usage exceeds replacement by 21 billion gallons a day.
- If you stop using flush toilets, you would save 13,000 gallons of water from being contaminated by your 165 gallons of excrement per year

HOW TO COMPOST YOUR SHIT (IN TEN EASY STEPS):

1. Obtain a few same-sized 5 gallon buckets with lids (check construction site dumpsters) and clean them out if you have to.
2. Go back to those dumpsters and get the scrap lumber. This is what you'll need to make your badass ne'er flushing toilet (see picture #1).
3. Find a source of raw sawdust (i.e. not from a woodshop or lumber store which may use pressure treated wood – which is HIGHLY toxic, the "treatment" being Cromated Copper Arsenate, CCA or arsenic for short), mulch, shredded newspaper, rotting wood chips, leaf mould, peat moss, grass clippings (watch out for chemically treated grass, like ChemLawn), or any organic cover material. Hardwood sawdust and wheat straw decompose the fastest. This will be what you cover your shit with, and it will prevent your composting toilet from smelling bad (see picture #2). Try to keep your toilet covered with the lid when you're not using it. Both of these things will keep flies, which you can now think of as 'disease vectors' that carry germs from poop to your dinner plates, off your shit. Don't you wish all it took were grass clippings to keep your slack-ass housemates away from your shit, too?
4. Call around and find either (and this is important) a food grade, or, better yet, a plastic 55-gallon drum with a lid. This can run you about $7, but could be free, especially behind bakeries. Just look around whenever you're done pulling out bagels and pastries from the dumpster. This is where you can do your composting; especially living in a city, where having a traditional compost pile might not be possible, or at least be pretty tricky.

PICTURE #1

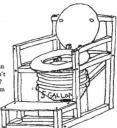

5-GALLON

5. Chop a hole in the lid to accept a length of ABS pipe (looks like black PVC, but is not PVC, which is one of the most toxic construction materials around). The pipe should be at least 1 foot long, and be split half in and half out of the drum lid. We speculate that if you had a long enough length, ran it to the bottom of the barrel, and drilled a bunch of ½" holes in it, the aeration would be way better and composting would be hastened. We haven't tried this method, so we don't know for sure. Cover the ends (or all the holes on the lower half) with bug screen (see picture #3). You now have your very own composter!

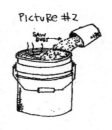

PICTURE #2

6. Piss and shit in your 5-gallon buckets. One bucket at a time, now. You have a few just in case you get lazy or totally drunk and pass out. As a starter, put 2-4" of you cover material on the bottom before your morning coffee, which we all know, gets them bowels movin'. Cover every "deposit" with a healthy can full of your cover material. In a punk house of four, this will fill up in 2 to 4 days, or thereabouts, depending on whether you eat anything besides bagels. Dump the full bucket into the 55-gallon drum, and occasionally roll the drum around. Yeah, yeah, we said don't turn your piles, but that's for an open-air, happy worm-with-the-munchies type pile. This is a closed 55-gallon drum with a little bit of airflow. This drum, by the way, gets left out in the sun, and it's a good idea to paint it black – you're an anarchist, dammit, and besides, the black absorbs heat really well and will probably heat up your crap to above 120 degrees Fahrenheit routinely (take a look at the dry ass charts again), probably killing anything dangerous throughout in one days time. If odors become a problem pee sometimes outside, on the soil, which can accept urine full strength. Don't pee on trees, the bark could burn, potentially compromising the health of the tree.

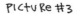

PICTURE #3

7. We would imagine you could also toss in kitchen scraps. With the proper carbon (which is what food scraps have a lot of)/nitrogen (which is what your crap has a lot of) ratio (the ideal being 30/1) you'll get what's called "thermophilic" conditions and the whole thing will easily heat up, without the sun, to over 120 degrees Fahrenheit and most likely stay that way for almost two weeks. Most backyard compost piles have little to no nitrogen, which is why they fuckin' fester and never seem to do much of anything, and smell like rotting nastiness (because that's exactly what it is). If you have a back yard and neighbors who aren't too pesky, including humanure with all it's bad-assed nitrogen is the ideal thing for your compost.

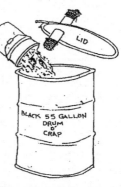

BLACK 55 GALLON
DRUM
O'
CRAP

8. Shit breaks down really fast. After the last dumping of the 5 gallon bucket into the drum (not quite totally full of shit), it should take maybe four months of sitting around to be pretty well composted (although, very little composting happens above 140 degrees Fahrenheit). Most likely though, if it's summertime, and if you've had some good sun days, the crap will be totally hygienic after a month. Eventually, you are going to want to give the good worms a chance at it. Good worms could be Arkansas Red Wigglers, or any old Earthworm, really. If you had outdoor composting, they'd just make their way over naturally and chow down on the "cooling phase" part of your pile.

9. It's time to part with your shit. Again, if you have any access to an outdoor compost pile, dump it there. There will be a good amount of nitrogen left, and a HUGE amount of "beneficial microorganisms" in there to get the rest of the pile composting quicker than hell. Otherwise, take it somewhere at night and bury it. Yeah, it sucks to not enjoy the benefits of your nutrient rich soil additive, but watch as things grow like mad in your midnight garden.

10. So, it may not be possible for you to have a 55-gallon drum anywhere. You live in an apartment with hundreds of people, perhaps. The option could be obtaining a lot of 5-gallon buckets, say a dozen or more depending on how many people will be using them, crap and pee in 'em as per instructions 1,2,3, and some of 6. When they fill up, leave them in a sunny spot, with the lids on tight, for about a month or two. They also have to get over 122 degrees Fahrenheit for at least a full day. They will not compost, as it is not an aerobic situation. But, the heat will anaerobically destroy harmful pathogens. Some people say let it sit for six months. They're scaredy-cats. If you have room for six months worth of 5-gallon buckets, go for it. Pathogens are weak, and unless you have worms (and you'll know) or are really sick, it's not that big of a deal. While you're waiting for the buckets to sit around long enough, organize everyone in your building complex into the first inner-U.S. composting toilet utilizing structure. After you've kept the buckets heating for however long (ok, ok, longer is better...) go back to #9, and bury it clandestine-style. It'll probably still look like shit, so be mindful of the pigs. No, none of this is ideal. But, at least this way you're not contributing to Global ruination, and are keeping your organic excrement in nature.

Information for this was stolen from The Humanure Handbook, by Joe Jenkins. A great book by all accounts. Also, there is our personal experience, as well as graphics from The Ghetto Garden (which includes a good deal of our personal experience). Turn shitting into an act of revolution!

Shit composting is a Garbage Liberation Front sanctioned form of resistance.

TO PEE OR NOT TO PEE?

"IF IT'S YELLOW, LET IT MELLOW. IF IT'S BROWN, FLUSH IT DOWN." THIS IS A RULE WE LIVE BY AT MY HOUSE — NEVER FLUSHING AFTER WE PEE AS A WAY TO CONSERVE WATER. BUT RECENTLY I'VE BEEN TAKING THINGS A STEP FURTHER. WHY EVEN PEE IN THE TOILET AT ALL? OUR URINE IS FILLED WITH LOTS OF EXCESS VITAMINS & MINERALS. PEE IS ONE OF EARTH'S GREAT FERTILIZERS, SO RATHER THAN FLUSHING IT AWAY INTO THE TOXIC ABYSS OF THE SEWER SYSTEM WHY NOT PUT IT TO USE? I PEE OUT IN OUR BACK YARD AS MUCH AS POSSIBLE, BUT DURING THE DAYTIME MOST OF OUR BACK YARD IS VISIBLE TO THE STREET & OUR NEIGHBORS SO RATHER THAN EXPOSING MYSELF

TO THE WORLD I'VE BEGUN TO KEEP A
"PEE BOTTLE" IN MY ROOM. IT'S JUST AN
OLD ORANGE JUICE BOTTLE THAT I KEEP
UNDER MY BED & RELIEVE MYSELF IN
WHEN I DON'T FEEL LIKE HEADING OUT
BACK. WHENEVER IT FILLS UP I GO
DUMP IT ON THE COMPOST PILE OR
ELSEWHERE AROUND THE YARD. I'VE HEARD
THAT PEEING ON COMPOST PILES IS GOOD,
BUT SOMETIMES I WONDER IF MAYBE TOO
MUCH PEE WOULD BE BAD SO I DON'T ALWAYS
DUMP IT THERE. ALSO PEE CONTAINS
AMMONIA, WHICH KILLS PLANTS, SO YOU
NEVER WANT TO PEE DIRECTLY ONTO THE
ROOTS OF ANYTHING. IF YOU PEE ONTO THE
GROUND OR IN COMPOST THE AMMONIA WILL
EVENTUALLY EVAPORATE JUST LEAVING THE
GOOD STUFF BEHIND. BUT THIS IS ALSO
WHAT MAKES PEE STINK, SO BE WARNED,
IF YOU PEE IN A BOTTLE TRY NOT TO LET
IT SIT IN THERE TOO LONG BEFORE DUMPING
IT OR ELSE WHEN YOU EVENTUALLY DO
OPEN IT YOU MAY DISCOVER THE INTENSE
"AROMAS" PEE IS CAPABLE OF. PEE-YOO!

I FIXED THE Faucet

IN OUR TUB

ONE DAY THE WATER PRESSURE FOR OUR HOT WATER IN THE SHOWER COMPLETELY DISAPPEARED. EVEN IF YOU TURNED THE KNOB FULLY ON ONLY A SMALL TRICKLE OF WATER CAME OUT. THOUGH THE HOT WATER DIDN'T WORK THE COLD WATER DID, & ALSO BOTH THE HOT & COLD WATER WORKED PERFECTLY FINE IN THE REST OF THE SINKS & FAUCETS THROUGHOUT THE HOUSE. BEING THAT IT WAS THE DEAD OF WINTER IT MADE FOR CHILLINGLY UNCOMFORTABLE SHOWERS. ALSO, NO MATTER HOW HARD WE TURNED THE KNOB TO TURN OFF THE WATER IT WOULD STILL LET OUT A NEVERENDING DRIP DRIP DRIP.

NOW, I'M NO PLUMBER, THE ONLY PLUMBING EXPERIENCE I HAVE IS WHEN I DISCONNECTED THE PIPE UNDER OUR BATHROOM SINK TO COLLECT GREYWATER. STILL, I KNEW I HAD TO DO SOMETHING TO FIX THE PROBLEM, SO I GOT A HOME REPAIR BOOK FROM THE LIBRARY, BUSTED OUT A COUPLE TOOLS, & SET TO WORK. THE FIRST STEP WAS TO TURN OFF THE WATER SUPPLY TO THE FAUCET. IN OUR HOUSE THE VALVE FOR DOING THIS IS RIGHT AT THE HOT WATER HEATER IN OUR KITCHEN, BUT IN YOUR HOUSE THERE MAY BE A VALVE IN YOUR BATHROOM OR MAYBE OUTSIDE AT YOUR WATER METER. JUST TRY TO FOLLOW THE PATH OF YOUR WATER PIPE AS IT SNAKES THROUGHOUT YOUR HOUSE & YOU'LL EVENTUALLY FIND IT. SO I TURNED THAT SUCKER OFF, WENT BACK TO THE BATHROOM & SURE ENOUGH THERE WAS NO WATER SUPPLY TO THE FAUCET. NOW I WAS READY TO OPEN THINGS UP WITHOUT GETTING SPRAYED WITH A FLOOD OF WATER LIKE IT HAPPENS IN THE MOVIES.

I LEARNED FROM MY LIBRARY BOOK THAT IF YOU TAKE OFF THE FAUCET KNOB THERE'S A LITTLE RUBBER STOPPER INSIDE. WHEN THE KNOB IS TURNED OFF THE RUBBER STOPPER IS CLAMPED DOWN HOLDING THE WATER BACK, BUT WHEN YOU TURN IT ON THE STOPPER LIFTS UP ALLOWING THE WATER TO FLOW. USUALLY WHEN A FAUCET HAS A DRIPPING PROBLEM IT'S BECAUSE THE STOPPER IS OLD & HAS CORRODED OR CRACKED & SO IT'S SLOWLY LETTING WATER THROUGH.

SO I TOOK OUT THE SCREW HOLDING THE KNOB ON & WITH A LITTLE WIGGLING & YANKING THE KNOB POPPED RIGHT OFF. BENEATH THE KNOB WAS A NUT I HAD TO UNSCREW SO WITH THE HELP OF MY TRUSTY WRENCH I SCREWED IT RIGHT OFF.

ONCE I GOT IT OFF I
REALIZED IT WASN'T
JUST A NUT BUT A
WHOLE KNOBBY,
SCREWY CONTRAPTION.
AND ON THE END OF
IT WAS THE RUBBER
STOPPER I WAS LOOKING FOR. I EXAMINED
THE STOPPER & IT LOOKED FINE TO ME, NO
KNICKS OR CRACKS. SO I LOOKED IN THE
HOLE WHERE THE KNOB USED TO BE & THERE
LIED THE PROBLEM - A PIECE OF TRASH
HAD COME UP THROUGH THE PIPES & WAS
BLOCKING THE FLOW OF WATER. IT WAS
SOME PLASTICKY, PAPERY STUFF SO I JUST
FISHED IT OUT, SCREWED EVERYTHING
BACK INTO PLACE, TURNED ON THE WATER
& TA DA! NO MORE DRIP & THE WATER FLOWED
FREELY. JUST SO YOU KNOW, IF THE PROBLEM
HAD ACTUALLY BEEN THE STOPPER I
COULD HAVE JUST TAKEN IT OFF, GONE TO
THE HARDWARE STORE & GOT A BRAND NEW
ONE FOR A FEW BUCKS & REPLACED IT. EASY,
RIGHT? SO DON'T LET YOUR FAUCETS DRIP,
WASTING WATER SHOULD BE A CRIME.

HOW I FIXED MY HARMONICA

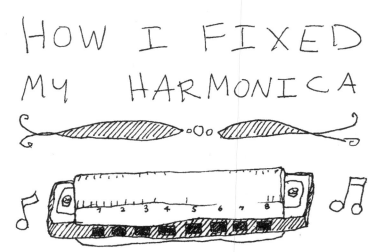

FOR A WHILE I WAS CARRYING MY HARMONICA WITH ME IN MY POCKET EVERYWHERE I WENT SO I WOULD ALWAYS BE PREPARED TO WHIP IT OUT & PRACTICE DURING ANY IDLE MOMENTS THROUGHOUT THE DAY. IT SEEMED LIKE A PRETTY GOOD IDEA, BUT WHAT I DIDN'T THINK ABOUT WAS THE FACT THAT LINT & OTHER DEBRIS TRAVELLED AROUND IN MY POCKET AS WELL. IT WAS ONLY A MATTER OF TIME BEFORE SOME OF IT FOUND ITS WAY INTO ONE OF THE HOLES IN MY HARMONICA, RENDERING IT MUSICALLY INEPT.

THE WAY I KNEW SOMETHING HAD
GONE AWRY IS THAT ONE OF THE
HOLES WHEN BLOWN INTO WOULD NO
LONGER PRODUCE A MUSICAL NOTE.
"THAT'S CURIOUS," I THOUGHT TO MY-
SELF, "I GUESS I'LL OPEN IT UP &
SEE WHAT'S THE TROUBLE."

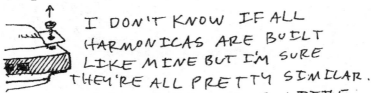

I DON'T KNOW IF ALL
HARMONICAS ARE BUILT
LIKE MINE BUT I'M SURE
THEY'RE ALL PRETTY SIMILAR.
SO I UNSCREWED THE 2 LITTLE
SCREWS ON EACH END OF THE HAR-
MONICA. THIS ALLOWED THE TOP
& BOTTOM METAL PIECES TO COME
OFF & LEFT ME WITH THE MIDDLE
PART WHICH IS WHAT I NEEDED.
IT LOOKS LIKE THIS:

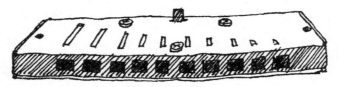

SORT OF.

SO ONCE AGAIN I JUST UN-
SCREWED THE SCREWS SO THAT
I COULD GET EVEN FURTHER
INTO THE INNARDS.

ONCE THE SCREWS ARE OUT IT
SEPARATES INTO 3 BASIC PARTS

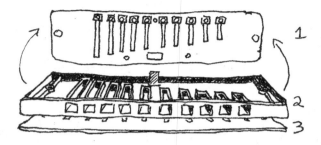

SEE THOSE 10 LITTLE THINGIES
HANGING DOWN ON PART #1?
WHEN YOU BLOW AIR INTO THE
HOLES OF THE HARMONICA IT
MAKES THOSE VIBRATE WHICH IS
WHAT MAKES THE SOUND. MY
PROBLEM WAS THAT A LITTLE
PIECE OF DEBRIS HAD LODGED
ITSELF UNDER ONE OF THOSE, SO
IT WAS UNABLE TO VIBRATE &
THUS MADE NO SOUND! SO I
JUST REMOVED THE INTRUDER
& THEN PUT EVERYTHING BACK
TOGETHER OPPOSITE OF THE WAY
I TOOK IT APART. I GAVE IT A
BLOW & IT SOUNDED LIKE NEW.
HOORAY!

DIY:
Fixing a
Broken Toilet

By Matte Resist

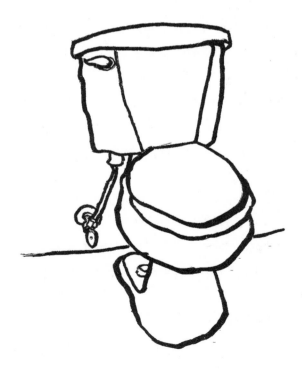

A broken toilet can be a constant source of aggravation. They run all day, and all night and you're constantly walking back to jiggle the handle to try to get it to stop. On top of that, a broken toilet wastes a lot of water. But you don't have to deal with that, cause I have recently discovered that toilets are about the easiest and cheapest things in your house to repair.

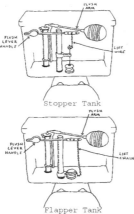

Stopper Tank

Flapper Tank

Generally the problem with the toilet is going to be the part I have highlighted red. There are a couple things to check before you mess with that though. First off, check the tank stopper (top left) or the flapper (bottom left) to see if it is in good condition. A deteriorated one will allow water to leak (making your toilet run constantly)

There are a ton of different types of stoppers, and my best suggestion would be, remember how you take it out. Bring it to the store with you, and get one that matches it exactly. Put it in.

Another thing to check is the chain. (bottom left only) When you flush the toilet, does the chain end up under the flapper? If so, you can either shorten the chain, or move the chain to a different hole on the trip lever. My toilet ran constantly! I moved the chain to the hole nearest the handle, and now it's fine! If the chain is twisted, it won't let the flapper down all the way. Just untwist it and reattach.

If your handle is getting stuck down, a little multi-purpose oil will often fix that. (not WD40!) If not, a new handle/flush lever can be purchased for about $2.50. All you have to do is disconnect the chain, remove one nut, slide the old one out, and put the new one in. Super Easy!

Last thing is the part I've highlighted red. These things will often look a lot different from the diagram. Probably brass with all kind of screws and moving parts. You can actually take that old one apart, replace rubber washers and whatnot, but usually that's just a short term solution. And for just $7, you can replace the whole assembly and not have to worry about it! For 75 cents more, you can replace the floater ball too. I would say that you could replace everything in your toilet for less than $15, and it's just like having a new toilet. You should never have to replace the toilet itself (unless one of your rowdy friends smashes it, or blows it up with a cherry bomb.)

At first glance, this may look like kind of an intimidating project. But it's really very easy! First look under the tank, and find the pipe that leads to it. It should have a handle on it. Turn that handle all the way in (so the water is off) Flush the toilet, holding the handle down until as much water as possible has drained. On the pipe you just turned off, there should be two nuts. One holds the flush assembly in the toilet, the other connects the water supply pipe to the flush assembly. Remove the supply nut first (a channel locks is your best bet, unless you have a large crescent or pipe wrench)

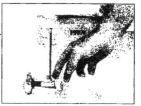

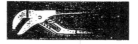

Next, remove the nut that is flush against the bottom of the tank. This will release the flush assembly. It would be a good idea to have a large bowl under the nut when you remove it, since there is probably still a good half a gallon of water that will come out as soon as you loosen the nut. Then just pull the old assembly straight out, and put the new one in. Most new ones can be adjusted for how much water you want in the tank, I usually set mine as low as possible to conserve water. When you put it back together, there should be rubber washers at each joint. Make sure to put them in, or you'll have water everywhere when you turn it back on. The last thing you need to do is connect the little hose to the top of the assembly. Just drop the other end into the hollow tube in the middle and turn the water back on.

BUILD YOUR OWN HOUSE (ON POISON HILL)(OR ANY PATCH OF NEGLECTED WOODS)

IT WAS OVER A YEAR AGO WHEN DAN HERMAN AND RYAN SET OUT TO BUILD SHACKS IN TOWN, OR RATHER, OUT ON THE EDGE. THEY FOUND A GREAT SPOT. IT'S BEST TO SCOPE YOUR FUTURE HOME OUT IN THE WINTER SO YOU KNOW HOW VISIBLE IT IS WHEN ALL THE LEAVES ARE GONE. SO ANY HOW, RYAN AND DAN H. LEFT TOWN, THEN A YEAR LATER CAME BACK TO BUILD. I GOT IN TOWN SOMETIME DECEMBER AND RYAN AND NAOMI WERE DONE WITH THEIRS. I BUILT MINE, THEN WHEN SPRING ROLLED AROUND, DAN H. SHOWED UP AND BUILT HIS. NOW THERE'S A GARDEN OUT THERE, AND A POND AND AN OUTDOOR KITCHEN. POISON HILL IS ALMOST IT'S OWN NEIGHBORHOOD NOW. THE IVY HAS TAKEN OVER, AND SO HAVE WE!!! AND SO COULD YOU!!! SICK OF RENT AND STUPID LANDLORDS AND TOILETS THAT KEEP BREAKING AND FAUCETS THAT DRIP? BUILD YOUR OWN HOUSE FROM TRASH! LIVE IN A SHACK!

HERE'S WHAT YOU'LL NEED — IT'S BEST TO START WITH SOME FRIENDS. TO MOTI-
VATE EACH OTHER TO SCAVENGE AND BUILD, BUT HECK, I SUPPOSE YOU COULD DO IT ALL BY YOUR SELF HERMIT STYLE. YOU'LL ALSO NEED THESE THINGS.....

- A SAW - TREES - NAILS - POTS - AN IRON SKILLET FOR COOKING - A KNIFE
- A HAMMER - - A TARP - - BLANKETS - - CARD BOARD - - PLASTIC - - -
- RANDOM SCRAPS OF WOOD - - SOME STRING - - WINDOWS ARE NICE - -

WITH GOOD IMAGINATION, ALL THESE THINGS ARE SUBJECT. THEY'RE WHAT I AND THE OTHER SHACK DWELLERS HAD TO WORK WITH, BUT REALLY, YOU CAN BUILD A SHACK WITH JUST ABOUT ANY THING.

HERE'S HOW I DID IT — FIRST I DUG THE FLOOR SOMEWHAT LEVEL.
NEXT I CUT 8 POSTS FROM FELLED PINE TREES THAT WERE ABOUT 6-8 INCHES DIAMETER. BURY THE POSTS ABOUT A FOOT DEEP, LEAVING 6-7 FEET OF POST STICKING UP, DEPENDING ON HOW TALL YOU ARE. THIS IS NOW THE FRAME FOR YOUR OUTSIDE WALLS, LIKE THIS.

PINE POSTS
FLOOR

NEXT, PUT PINE POSTS (OR ANY WOOD REALLY) ALL AROUND THE TOP, LIKE SO.

FRAME
PINE POSTS
FLOOR

ARGHH, I WILL ROT YO SKIN!

EMBRACE THEE POISON IVY

STAPLE CARD BOARD AND PLASTIC ON THE SIDES, PUT IN A WINDOW, INS-ULATE THE INNER WALLS WITH BLANKETS, THROW A TARP ON THE TOP, USE A BLANKET FOR THE DOOR, STURDY THE WALLS WITH STRING & NAILS, AND NEXT THING YA KNOW, YOU'RE HOME!

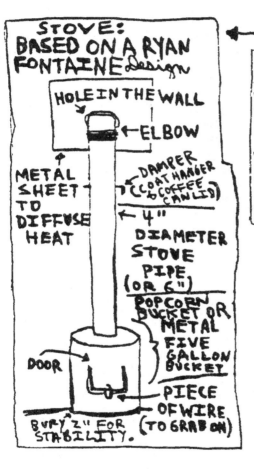

STOVE:
BASED ON A RYAN
FONTAINE Design

HOLE IN THE WALL

← ELBOW

METAL
SHEET
TO
DIFFUSE
HEAT

DAMPER
(COAT HANGER
& COFFEE
CAN LID)

← 4"

DIAMETER
STOVE
PIPE
(OR 6")

POPCORN
BUCKET OR
METAL
FIVE
GALLON
BUCKET

DOOR

PIECE
OF WIRE
(TO GRAB ON)

BURY 2" FOR
STABILITY.

ALL THIS YOU CAN DUMP
STER OR GET AT A HARD
WARE STORE. IF YOU
HAVENT A CHISEL, YOU CAN
CUT THE HOLE IN THE
STEEL WALL (AND THE
DOOR AND STOVE PIPE
HOLE IN THE BUCKET)
WITH A SCREWDRIVER
AND HAMMER
P.S. BUILD FIRES SMALL
AT FIRST AND BEWARE
OF TOXINS IN
FIVE GALLON CAN.

How to Do Basic Electrical Wiring
Joe Biel

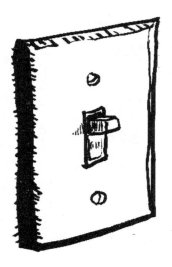

Electrical wiring is really basic and simple. It can also be very safe when taking the proper precautions and with a basic understanding of conductivity.

Electricity works through a series of conductors and resistors. Metal is a conductor whereas cloth and rubber are resistors. This is why pliers have rubber handles and why your electrical wires are wrapped in rubber sheathing.

You'll need a few basic tools to begin. Needle nose and lineman's pliers are pretty essential, as are a circuit tester and screwdriver. First, you'll want to make sure that your circuit isn't live when you're working on it. You can do this in your home by turning off the appropriate switch in the breaker box. You must also check that the circuit is actually turned off by taking your circuit tester and putting one lead on the white wire and one lead on the black wire. If the light doesn't come on, your circuit is dead. If it is lit, then there is still electricity traveling through the circuit and you shut off the wrong one.

Electricity wants to take the shortest and easiest path to the ground. The setup of a wiring diagram tries to create that path, but sometimes, when you contact live wires, the shortest path will unfortunately be through your body. This is why it is essential to make sure the power is off. *Never touch positive and negative live wires at the same time!*

Most homes have either 2 or 3 wire systems. If you open up an electrical box and you find two different wires then the dark one is the positive (carries electricity from the source) and the white one is the negative (sends electricity back to the source). Sometimes, in older homes, enough dirt and dust collects that you have to clean off the sheathing to tell which wire is which. This is safe as long as you don't touch the exposed parts of the wires.

If there's a third wire with green sheathing or no sheathing at all then that's a ground wire. That's the wire that keeps the circuit grounded to something metal to prevent the wire from kicking the breaker if it's overloaded. It's also present for safety.

If there's a fourth red wire, then that means the circuit is a little more complicated. This is a second positive wire for wiring something like a switch or complex. Consult a book from your library when needing to rewire one of these circuits. Otherwise, just put it back the same way that you found it when replacing a switch or receptacle.

All wiring is done inside little plastic or metal boxes. This is done for safety reasons, to prevent fires, and so that your live current is not where someone could accidentally touch a live circuit and electrocute themselves. If you split up an existing box or add a new circuit along a line, be sure to put everything inside a box. You'll just want to screw it into a wall stud or ceiling joist.

Most wiring problems result from work that was done improperly in the past or from hardware wearing out. It takes quite a few years for hardware to wear out, so generally you'll be dealing with fixing half-assed jobs or human error. With that in mind, take the time to do things right and keep it clean.

When you first open up an unfamiliar box, just take the time to find out where all the lines come from and go to. Trace it back to the source and understand how your power grid works. Think of ways that the setup could be more efficient. This will come more naturally with time. Look at all the wires and connections inside the box. Generally, black wires will be connected to other black wires and white wires connected to other white wires. These are the most basic kinds of circuits and a good starter to understanding the way current works.

When you add a new part to a circuit or change an existing circuit the first thing you want to do is shut down the power and make sure that circuit is not live with your electrical tester. After that you should disconnect the black positive wires and point them away from each other. Next, disconnect the white wires and do the same. Finally, disconnect the ground wire if there is one. If you are adding a receptacle (outlet) to the box, you'll attach the black wire to the copper (darker) side of the receptacle, and the white wire to the chrome (lighter) side. If there is a ground wire, it screws into the bottom. Attach new wires in the reverse of the order you disconnected them – ground, then white, then black.

Reattach the existing wires and your new wire by taking your lineman's pliers and making all the wires straight. Hold them together in the pliers and twist them all together in a clockwise motion. This will make it much easier to keep things neat and tidy. Make sure to put wire caps (little plastic caps available at a hardware store) onto the finished, twisted wires. This prevents your positives and negatives from contacting each other inside the box, which can cause electrical fires. Sometimes you'll encounter old cloth sheathing on your wires. If it's fraying, you'll want to trim down the excess cloth before putting them back together.

Sometimes, when you're working with older wires, you'll encounter aluminum wires. You won't want to attach modern copper wires to these, but rather, replace the old aluminum with copper back to the source. Another problem you may run into is older wires becoming brittle and cracking when you take them apart. You may have to strip the wires back further and attempt to reattach them. Just be slow and cautious.

Turn on your power. If something is wired incorrectly, it will most likely blow your fuse or breaker right away, but if you check things carefully and move slowly and cautiously, you should prevent things like that before turning the power back on. Check your circuit. Are all the connections good? If there is a receptacle, is it getting power? You can also get a plug in tester to make sure everything is wired properly in a receptacle.

Hopefully, after working on a few different circuits, you will build up confidence to work on more complicated projects. Eventually you'll be able to rewire projects in the most organized and efficient manner.

SOLAR
COMPOSTING TOILET → a bathroom fixture used for defecation and urination
↳ A mixture of various decomposing organic substances such as leaves, manure, etc. used for fertilizing land.

A composting toilet treats sewage by decomposing it into a rich soil. Decomposition is achieved by the action of bacteria in the presence of:

1. AIR   2. WARMTH (50-150°F)   3. MOISTURE

DECOMPOSITION OF SEWAGE SERVES THREE PURPOSES:
(all of them worthy!)

1. Takes away the ODOR & UGLINESS OF SHIT

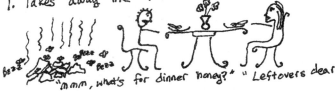

"mmm, what's for dinner honey?" "Leftovers dear"

2. Saves nutrients in sewage for reuse as fertilizer

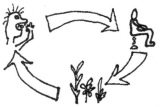

A family of six produces enough nutrients in a year to grow 3000 lbs (!!) of vegetables. Think about this amazing fact!

3. The plant nutrients are retained in a form in which they are easily used by plants but not so easily washed out of soil and into ground water or run off, where they're considered pollution.

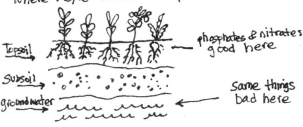

Topsoil

Subsoil

groundwater

phosphates & nitrates good here

same things bad here

PATHOGENS & PASTEURIZATION:

↳ disease causing organisms (often bacteria)

↳ exposing a substance to heat at a certain temperature for a certain length of time to destroy disease causing organisms.

THERE MIGHT BE PATHOGENS IN HUMAN SHIT. IF THESE PATHOGENS ARE NOT DESTROYED ~~BEFORE~~ THE SHIT IS USED TO FERTILIZE VEGETABLE CROPS THEN THE FOLLOWING HEALTH AFFLICTIONS MAY BE SPREAD: diarrhea, cholera, hookworm, roundworm, hepatitis A, and more!

THERE SEEMS TO BE A MISUNDERSTANDING OVER WHETHER OR NOT COMPOSTING HUMAN SHIT KILLS PATHOGENS. THE ANSWER SEEMS TO BE THAT WHILE COMPOSTING MAY DESTROY SOME PATHOGENS, IT DOES NOT GUARANTEE ALL PATHOGEN DESTRUCTION. PASTEURIZATION IS THE GUARANTEED WAY TO DESTROY PATHOGENS.

BEEEB
FLY + HAND + MOUTH =

the way pathogens are transmitted from shit to healthy humans.

Regardless of the sewage treatment method, if flies are getting into and out of the "Shithole", there is a potential health threat.

PASTEURIZATION TAKES: 2 WEEKS AT 113° F (45°C)   the higher the
24 HOURS AT 122° F (50°C)   temperature the
30 MINUTES AT 149° 5 (65°C)   less time it takes

TWO INTERESTING THINGS TO NOTICE ARE:

1. A good compost pile will self-heat (because the process of decomposition is exothermic, or liberates heat) and can reach 100°F – 140°F. So it is possible that a compost pile will pasteurize itself. The problem is that the inside of the pile gets hot but the outside stays cool, and the pathogens might be anywhere!

2. 122°F → 149°F are temperatures easily reached in passive solar heaters. A well insulated box with a window that faces the sun can easily maintain 149°F for a few hours on a sunny day.

some commercial composting toilets use an electric heater. gosh, that gets expensive!

SOME NOTES ON COMPOST:

BEFORE BUILDING A COMPOSTING TOILET SOME EXPERIENCE WITH COMPOST PILES IS HELPFUL. MOST SERIOUS GARDENERS REVERE THEIR COMPOST PILES WITH RELIGIOSITY AND MYSTIC ENTHUSIASM SO TALKING TO GARDENERS CAN BE EDUCATIONAL (AND ENTERTAINING). THERE ARE ALSO MANY GOOD BOOKS ON COMPOSTING.

"...then i mix in a cup of bone meal and a handful of rusty nails, i don't turn it again until the full moon and i only water it with rain water collected off the shed roof... Sometimes when it starts to warm up i just kind of sit by it on those chilly october mornings..."

I think the reason people become so obsessed with compost is that it's one of the few processes in nature where you end up with more than you started with, sort of like alchemy, the belief that if you mix wheat chaff and old rags with the right porportion of bronze filings you get pure GOLD. Find out for yourself...

IN GENERAL, COMPOST PILES LIKE 5 THINGS:

1. CRITICAL MASS
The bigger a compost pile is, the better it works.

2. WARMTH 50°F-120°F (Although composting can occur up to 150°F) too cold and there is not enough biological activity. too hot and the bacteria are killed.

3. AIR composting bacteria are AEROBIC they like AIR (the oxygen in AIR)
Air can get into a pile through cracks and openings formed by twigs and straws. People also "turn" or "fluff up" the pile with a pitchfork.

4. MOISTURE H_2O. JUST ENOUGH BUT NOT TOO MUCH.
When dry, a pile must be watered. During rainy periods it may have to be covered with a tarp. The larger the pile, the less one needs to worry about moisture.

5. BALANCE OF CHEMICALS
40 carbon : 1 Nitrogen
carbon is like dry leaves nitrogen is like fish guts.
human shit is about 30C:1N

SOME NOTES ON URINE (PEE)

URINE DOES NOT TRANSMIT PATHOGENS IN THE NORTHERN HEMISPHERE. SO PEE WHERE YOU PLEASE.

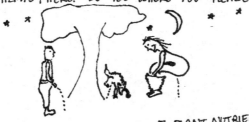

SINCE PEE IS A GREAT SOURCE OF PLANT NUTRIENTS, it IS DESIRABLE TO SAVE PEE FOR THE PLANTS BY PEEING IN THE COMPOST PILE.

SINCE THOSE SAME NUTRIENTS ARE CONTAMINANTS IN GROUNDWATER, LAKES, AND STREAMS, IT IS GOOD TO PEE IN THE COMPOST PILE, AND NOT IN A STREAM.

PEE CAN BE ADDED DIRECTLY TO ANY COMPOSTING TOILET, BUT TOO MUCH PEE CAN MAKE THE COMPOST TOO WET (SWAMPY).

PEE CAN BE COLLECTED IN A CONTAINER AND ADDED TO THE COMPOST PILE WHEN IT IS CONVENIENT, BUT THIS SHOULD BE DONE OFTEN, AS OLD PEE STARTS TO STINK.

ONCE my friend collected 5 gallons of urine in his room. He was transporting it to the first floor to dump it in the toilet when he was distracted and put the bucket down. A week later somebody knocked the bucket over. The lid popped off and pee went everywhere, seeping through the floor and eventually raining down in the kitchen from the ceiling! To make matters worse, he was out of town on vacation when the spill occured. Needless to say, the accident made him temporarily unpopular among the house mates. Infact, his name is still cursed on humid july afternoons.

Our composting toilet has a pee drain where extra pee drains into a homemade charcoal filter just below the ground. Much of the pee is absorbed by the straw, and toilet paper. I usually just pee directly into the compost pile or under a tree.

MIX PEE WITH 6X WATER TO ADD DIRECTLY UNDER PLANTS

DETAILS OF OUR SOLAR COMPOSTING TOILET.
OUR SYSTEM CAN BE THOUGHT OF AS HAVING 3 STAGES:
1. COLLECTION   2. PASTEURIZATION   3. COMPOSTING.

Because we scavenged and bartered many of our materials, and the dimensions are very flexible, what follows shows show things are done + how they could be done. This way others can adapt the design to make use of local resources and conditions.

I. COLLECTION :

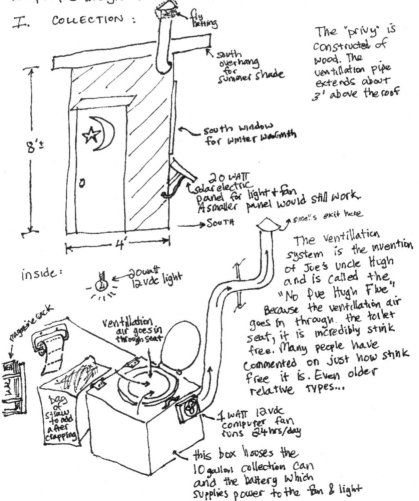

fly netting

south overhang for summer shade

The "privy" is constructed of wood. The ventilation pipe extends about 3' above the roof

south window for winter warmth

8' ±

20 WATT solar electric panel for light + fan. A smaller panel would still work.

SOUTH

4'

smell's exit here

The ventillation system is the invention of Joe's uncle Hugh and is called the "No fue Hugh Flue". Because the ventillation air goes in through the toilet seat, it is incredibly stink free. Many people have commented on just how stink free it is. Even older relative types...

inside:

20 watt 12 vdc light

magazine rack

ventillation air goes in through seat

bag of straw to add after crapping

4 WATT 12 vdc computer fan runs 24 hrs/day

this box houses the 10 gallon collection can and the battery which supplies power to the fan & light

THE BOX THAT HOUSES THE 10 GALLON COLLECTION CAN
IS BUILT SORT OF CAREFULLY SO THAT IT CAN BE
OPENED FOR EASY ACCESS TO THE CAN, BUT SO THAT
FLIES AND BUGS CANNOT GET IN THROUGH CRACKS.
THE FAN RUNS ALL THE TIME, DRAWING AIR THROUGH THE
TOILET SEAT HOLE. FLIES DO NOT ENTER THROUGH
THIS HOLE BECAUSE THE CONSTANT NEGATIVE PRESSURE
PREVENTS SMELLS FROM GETTING OUT, AND FLIES
ARE ATTRACTED BY SMELLS (even though they have
96 eyes, flies are attracted by smell, go figure...) FLIES
MAY GATHER AROUND THE TOP OF THE VENTILLATION STACK,
BUT THE POSITIVE AIR PRESSURE AND SCREEN PREVENTS THEM
FROM GETTING IN. THE DIMENSIONS OF THE BOX WILL VARY
DEPENDING ON THE DIMENSIONS OF YOUR CAN.

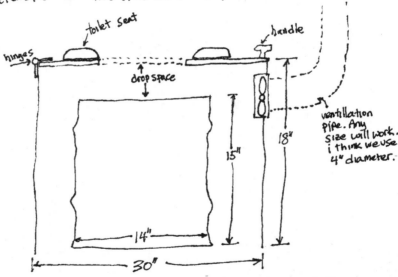

LEAVE PLENTY OF ROOM IN THE BOX TO REACH IN AND
REMOVE THE HEAVY CAN. OUR BOX ALSO STORES
THE 12 VOLT, 50 AMP-hour DEEP CYCLE BATTERY
WHICH STORES ELECTRICITY TO POWER THE FAN
(A LITTLE ONE WATT BOX FAN OFF OF AN OLD COMPUTER.)
AND THE LIGHTBULB (A 12VDC 20W -75W BULB,
A TAIL LIGHT BULB OFF A CAR WOULD WORK.)

SOME NOTES ON THE SIZE OF THE COLLECTION CAN

We collect shit in 10 gallon cans, 15" high and 14" in diameter. With three people and guests using the shitter, we need to change cans about every two weeks. We mix a little straw on top of each "solid waste visit". The straw increases the carbon ratio, absorbs extra pee, creates a conduit for air, absorbs smells, and is aesthetically pleasing. You could use any size can. Some use 55 gallon drums. The advantage of a 55g. drum is you can compost right in it, and have a good chance of pasteurization. The problems are:

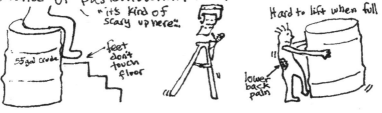

"it's kind of scary up here".

55 gal crude

feet don't touch floor

Hard to lift when full

lower back pain

THE LARGER SIZE OF THE 55 GALLON DRUM ALSO MAKES IT HARDER TO HEAT UP. IT IS MORE DIFFICULT TO USE SOLAR ENERGY TO ENSURE THAT THE ENTIRE CONTENTS HAVE PASTEURIZED. FOR (see next page) THE 10 GALLON CAN WE BUILT A SMALL, DISCRETE INSULATED BOX. A NORMAL PROBE THERMOMETER EASILY REACHES THE MIDDLE OF THE CAN TO INDICATE TEMPERATURE BEING REACHED. THE FIRST SUNNY DAY ALWAYS PASTEURIZES THE CONTENTS.

IF ONE WANTED TO PUT THE COLLECTION CAN AND BOX IN A NORMAL SIZE INDOOR BATHROOM, A 10 gallon CAN FITS EASILY. A 55 GALLON DRUM IN THE BATHROOM MIGHT PROVE CUMBERSOME.

our 10 gallon cans were obtained from army surplus for $3.00 (with lids)

YOU WILL NEED 2 CANS, SO WHILE ONE IS IN THE PASTEURIZER THE OTHER IS IN THE COLLECTION BOX GETTING FILLED UP.

II PASTEURIZATION:

When the collection bucket in the privy is full, it is removed and placed in a pasteurizer.

solar glazing

insulated box

Collection can getting hot

OUR SOLAR PASTEURIZER IS AN OLD SCAVENGED INSULATING COVER FOR A SOLAR HOT WATER HEATER STORAGE TANK. THE OUTSIDE IS THICK SUNLIGHT RESISTANT PLASTIC, THE INSIDE IS 4" THICK POLYEUROTHANE INSULATION.

FOR SOLAR GLAZING WE USED A PIECE OF GREENHOUSE PLASTIC, (TRANSPARENT POLYCARBONATE)

FOR THE BOX, ANY WELL INSULATED AND WEATHER TIGHT BOX WILL WORK (AN OLD SMALL REFRIGERATOR TURNED ON ITS BACK?)

FOR GLAZING, GLASS OR PLASTIC IS FINE, ANY OLD WINDOW, GOOD.

THE THING HAS TO TILT TO ADJUST TO THE SEASONAL CHANGES IN THE SUNS ALTITUDE.

YOU NEED TO PLACE IT SOMEWHERE IN THE YARD OR ON THE ROOF WHERE IT GETS GOOD SUNLIGHT EXPOSURE.

3½" OF FIBREGLASS INSULATION OR ITS EQUIVALENT (CARDBOARD, STRAW)

GET AN OLD SOUP THERMOMETER FROM A USED RESTAURANT SUPPLY PLACE TO CHECK TEMP..

WHEN THE PASTEURIZER GETS HOT IT HAS A TENDENCY TO STINK FOR A COUPLE HOURS. OURS SITS IN THE MIDDLE OF THE YARD AND WE IGNORE IT, BUT YOU MIGHT WANT TO LOCATE YOURS OUT BACK, AT LEAST 25' FROM THE NEIGHBORS HOUSE AND DOWNWIND. OR TRY A VENT STACK?

The solar pasteurizer is like a very hot cold frame, or a cool solar cooker. However, i do not recommend using it for cooking nor growing plants!

III. COMPOSTING

Once pasteurized, the now harmless but probably ugly and still aromatic mixture of straw, piss, shit, and toilet paper is added to the center of a large regular compost pile, someplace the neighborhood dogs and the neighborhood Association won't go digging in it.

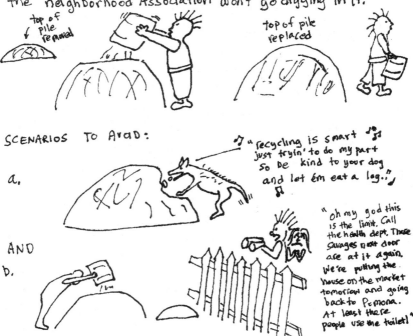

top of pile removed

top of pile replaced

SCENARIOS TO AVOID:

a.

♪ "recycling is smart just tryin' to do my part so be kind to your dog and let 'em eat a log." ♪

AND

b.

"oh my god this is the limit. Call the health dept. These savages next door are at it again. We're putting the house on the market tomorrow and going back to Pomona. At least these people use the toilet!"

Assuming you CAN prevent scenarios (a) & (b), come springtime you will have the greatest compost anywhere available. We are also experimenting with using a worm box to compost the pasteurized sewage. The small size and high efficiency of a worm box might be good for urban situations.

HAPPY SHITING!

Dirty, Dirty World.

Betcha didn't know that (literally) thousands of the everyday chemicals in our environment work synergistically in your body to alter your nervous, reproductive, and endocrine systems. Scary, eh? If you want to reduce your overall toxic exposure, if you suffer from Multiple Chemical Sensitivity (MCS) or have allergic reactions to common household items, keep reading. Not just industrial pollutants like dioxin, but household stuff like cleaners and textiles can seriously screw with your body and even change your behavior, intelligence, fertility, and physiology. If you suffer from chronic conditions like depression/irritability, rashes, frequent headaches or migraines, learning difficulties, dark circles under your eyes, and/or joint pain that your doctor can't explain or help, you're probably chemically sensitive. Consult an environmental health specialist and start to reduce your toxic exposure with some simple changes. In this handy pull-out is a bunch of easy recipes to help break your chemical addiction to household cleaners. For more info and more resources, check out the reading list that follows.

This is not an exhaustive list. There are way more poisonous cleaners out there and way more easy ways to replace them. Doing so will improve your health and save you a LOT of money, cause you know this crap is expensive! You can also buy safer products in bulk at your health food store – bring your own container and save a lot.

1. Get rid of household poisons. Anything with a skull and crossbones or the words DANGER, POISON, WARNING or CAUTION on the label is dangerous and should be thrown out. Dispose of this stuff properly at your town's household hazardous waste site.

2. Assemble a nontoxic cleaning kit. You can do ALL your cleaning with the following items: a spray bottle of 50/50 vinegar and water, liquid soap (like Dr. Bronner's)* – NOT DETERGENT, and a can of NON-CHLORINE scouring powder. Gawd it's that easy. Other stuff you can use are baking soda, salt, borax (look in the laundry aisle at the supermarket), distilled white vinegar, and lemon juice.

*Make your own liquid soap: mix 2 cups grated bar soap w/ 1 gallon water in a pot, and stir over low heat until water boils and soap dissolves. Lower heat and simmer 10 minutes. Cool and store.

The following pull-out section is for you to stick in your cabinet or someplace you can refer to it. Please feel free to photocopy & share w/ your friends!

... be healthy!

Drain cleaner (like Liquid Plumr): lye poisoning can cause irreperable harm, plus drain cleaners just don't work too well. Use a drain strainer to keep food and crap from going down there. The best way to get rid of a big clog is with a plunger — no joke! A few plunges usually breaks up the clog quite well. For preventive measures or slow drains, pour 1 handful baking soda and 1/2 cup white vinegar down the drain and cover tightly. A fizzy reaction will dislodge small clogs and keep drains flowing freely.

Ammonia/ all-purpose cleaners (like Mr. Clean): very harmful to skin, eyes and lungs, can exacerbate asthma. Make your own all-purpose cleaner by mixing 1 tsp. liquid soap into 1 qt. warm water. Add some lemon juice or vinegar to cut grease. This solution will do for almost all your household cleaning needs.

Mold & mildew cleaners (like Formula 409): possible carcinogens, strong irritant to eyes, throat, skin & lungs. Instead mix borax and water or vinegar in a spray bottle. Spray it on and wipe mold off. You can use heat to kill a major mold problem: put a cheap electric heater in the room, turn it up high, close the door, and let it bake all day or overnight. The mold dries up into a powder that brushes off. You can use a hair dryer for smaller areas.

Lysol & other disinfectants: danger of poisoning by both ingestion and inhalation. Can damage liver, kidneys, lungs, and other organs, including the central nervous system (symptoms include depression and irritability). That "fresh clean smell" is actually nerve poison. Some joke, huh? Most of the time you don't even need a disinfectant, and if you do, soap and hot water is the best one there is. For large areas like floors, use a solution of 1/2 cup borax dissolved in 1 gallon hot water.

Glass cleaners (like Windex): irritating fumes and eye damage are the big problems here (see the ammonia section). Use 50/50 water and vinegar in a spray bottle, wipe off with a rag. Regular glass cleaner leaves a gooey residue that may show up as streaks the first time you use the nontoxic stuff. It will go away after the second cleaning.

Silver polish & other metal cleaners: contain ammonia, as well as petroleum distillates; varying toxicity. Did you know that you can magnetize tarnish away? You need some salty water and something aluminum (a pot, pan, or aluminum foil all work fine). Submerge the tarnished thing in the salty water with the aluminum thing, and then wipe dry after a few minutes. Badly tarnished items may need more than one trip through. This is a great magic trick when babysitting.

be clean...

Furniture & floor polish (like Mop&Glo): These contain carcinogenic phenols (very dangerous!!) and highly toxic nitrobenzine. Exposure during use & residual fumes are both dangerous. Aerosol sprays are particularly harmful because you will almost certainly inhale it during use. Instead, use mineral oil and apply sparingly with a soft cloth. You can add some lemon juice to get the nice smell. Almost any oil will clean and condition wood, including olive & vegetable oils. Polish when dry with a chamois cloth.

Rug, carpet & upholstery shampoo: contain dangerous solvents that can do both short- and long-term damage to the central nervous system. They leave residues in the textile that give off toxic vapors. Use plain baking soda to deodorize your carpets: get a big box and sprinkle VERY liberally all over the carpet. Let it sit at least 15 minutes and then vacuum up. Wipe up spills immediately to avoid stains. A good spot remover is a solution of 1/4 cup borax dissolved in 2 cups cold water, undiluted vinegar, or lemon juice.

Air fresheners (like Glade): these are usually either strong perfumes or chemicals that deaden your nerves so you can't detect the offending odor. Great idea, eh? Open the window, turn on a fan, take out the garbage, clean up food messes, empty the cat box, do your laundry... forget the fruity-smelling nerve agents. If you really want a nice fancy smell use some fresh-cut flowers or herbs from your garden! Check out the big jars of bulk herbs and flowers at your health food store and make a nice (and cheap) little sachet or potpourri. You can improve indoor air quality without poisoning yourself or spending money.

More tips: Don't use anything called "detergent" -- use soap instead. Health food stores are great resources for nontoxic household stuff, and you can usually save a LOT of money by refilling big containers at the store (it's even cheaper than the toxic stuff you're used to). Get yourself some Dr. Bronner's liquid soap!! For mail-order sources, check out the internet.

A word on pesticides: everyday household stuff like Round-up, Spectracide, and Raid are powerful toxins that kill humans and wildlife just the same as insects and weeds. Short-term exposure can cause illness, inflammation, hemorrhaging, headaches, nausea, fatigue, irritability, weight loss and depression. But think of how many toxics you've been exposed to through your lifetime. Long-term exposure causes cancer, birth defects, reproductive disorders, and a host of other chronic (and sometimes fatal) problems. You can find safer ways to deal with minor inconveniences like dandelions or ants. Check out the reading list and visit www.beyondpesticides.org for more information.

Household Tips and Lessons to be Learned

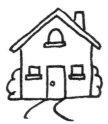

• If you get petroleum jelly on fabric, before laundering or having it cleaned, try rubbing talcum powder into it. You have to rub, rub, rub, but sometimes it will remove all of the petroleum jelly.

• If you have a bag of fiberfill - the kind used for stuffed animals - then you have a spare pillow when you need one. Just slip the entire bag into a pillowcase and it's ready for use. This is good for travel pillows, too.

• Those glass or plastic measuring bowls or pitchers that measure more than one cup at a time can be expensive. Just use pint or quart jars; some are even marked with ounces and cups.

WHAT DO YOU DO WITH . . .

. . . those *powdered cereal crumbs* in the bottom of the bag?
◊   Add them to muffins or pancakes in place of some of the flour
◊   Mix them with ground beef when making hamburgers, meatballs or meatloaf.
◊   Mix them in bread, biscuit or tortilla dough. Either use them to replace part of the flour or add more liquid to the recipe.
◊   Sprinkle them on top of ice cream or pudding.
◊   Thicken soup and stew with them.
◊   Add them to granola, hot cereal or rice pilaf.
◊   Replace some of the graham cracker crumbs in pie crust with them.
Consider whether your crumbs are from sweetened or unsweetened cereal before you use them. In some things it won't matter but you won't want to thicken soup with sugary crumbs.

. . . *syrup* from canned fruits and leftover juice, kool-aid or other fruit or fruit flavored drinks?
◊   Mix the syrup with the last of the fruit drink. You can pour it into small cups now and freeze with a spoon, bowl side down in it, for popsicles. This is really very sugary, so at this point I add water till it tastes right

. . . *the stalks* from fresh broccoli?
◊   If the skin is very tough, peel it off. Cut the tender insides into broccoli sticks to eat like carrot sticks, or cook them the same way you cook the florets.

. . . *the paper bags* sugar and flour come in?
◊   Reheat dinner rolls in them. Put the rolls in the bag, fold the top closed, run water over the bag and put in a 200 to 250 degree oven for 10 minutes or so.
◊   Use them to wrap glassware in for storage or moving.
◊   Use them for kitchen compost or garbage collectors. When they're full, close them up and toss them in the compost pile or dispose of them however you need to.
◊   stuff them with waste paper and/or small sticks, smash them flat and use them as fire starters.

. . . *old newspapers?*
◊   Use them for mulch in the garden.
◊   Peel vegetables or fruits onto them. When finished, pull the four corners together and dispose of the whole package.
◊   Line drawers or shelves with them. Tape in place using as little tape as possible for easy removal when the paper gets dirty. This is great for high up places that you normally wouldn't notice. When they get good and dusty, just fold them up and replace them with clean paper.
◊   Wrap gifts with them.
◊   Fold them into hats for kids

THIS SUMMER, LIKE MOST, WAS HOT... REALLY, REALLY HOT. WITH THE HEAT OF THE SEASON CAME THE OH SO FAMILIAR BUGS OF SUMMER. THERE WERE THE BUGS THAT WE DIDN'T MIND SO MUCH (MAYBE EVEN ENJOYED) LIKE JUNEBUGS AND CRICKETS. UNFORTUNATELY THERE WERE ALSO THE TORMENTORS - FLEAS, MOSQUITOS, AND FLIES. THIS SUMMER, EVERY NEW PIECE OF PRODUCE BROUGHT INTO OUR HOUSE SEEMED TO BE A SACCHARIN MATING CALL TO ONE PARTICULARLY ANNOYING BREED - THE FRUIT FLY. THESE THINGS WERE SUCH PROLIFIC BREEDERS, THAT A WEEK OF NEGLECT OF OUR OWN PERSONAL POPULATION WOULD ENSURE THE INFILTRATION OF THESE BUZZING BOTHERS IN EVERY CRANNY OF OUR SPACIOUS PAD - NOT JUST THE KITCHEN, BUT THE BATHROOM AND BEDROOMS AS WELL. NOT ONLY DID THEY GROSS US OUT, BUT IT WAS HARD TO PASS THEM OFF AS PETS WHEN WE ENTERTAINED, "HERE'S YOUR BEER, PAL, BUT LET ME FISH THAT FLY OUT FOR YOU FIRST." DETERMINED TO MINIMIZE THE PRESENCE OF THE FLYING MOOCHERS IN OUR HOUSEHOLD, I DID SOME RESEARCH, AND COMPILED SOME INFO ON HOW TO TRAP, KILL, OR DETER THE PESTS. I SPENT A COUPLE WEEKS PUTTING EACH METHOD TO THE TEST SO THAT I COULD SHARE WITH YOU THE RESULTS OF MY EXPERIMENTS ON

HOW TO GET RID OF FRUIT FLIES

THE MOST IMPORTANT THING TO DO IS TO FIGURE OUT WHERE THEY ARE COMING FROM (WHERE THEY ARE MAKIN' BABIES). MY FLIES WERE VERY ELUSIVE - I NEVER REALLY FOUND EVIDENCE OF ONE DISTINCT FLY HATCHING EPICENTER, BUT I DID THE FOLLOWING THINGS TO SORT OF COVER ALL THE BASES.

① Check to see if they are coming from a sink drain. Fruit flies need a source of moisture and food to reproduce - this makes a seldomly used sink drain the perfect place. To check this possibility,

You can put plastic wrap over the drain pipe and tape it down. Wait a day or so to see if little flies appear trapped under the plastic. If so, this might be the fly nursery. Scrub the inside of the drain if possible or rinse it with a blast of high pressure water if you have a spray nozzle fixture on your sink. You can also slowly pour boiling water down the sides of the drain to dislodge any larvae. YUCK! Once done, remember to use the offending drain more often—getting water to run through it more regularly will prevent the flies from settling in.

② Look for maggots (tiny rice looking things that wiggle) in wet caulking around your sink or tub. Clean these areas and dry them thoroughly. Check any wet dishtowels or sponges. If they might be a nesting site – boil them and let them dry. Look for any drips under the sink or behind the fridge that might be creating a suitable breeding climate for flies and remedy these types of problems.

③ Take out your trash more frequently. Flies love to linger and breed in the soupy mess that sometimes collects at the bottom of your trash bag. Move organic kitchen wastes outside and compost them: you will be recycling; your soil will thank you, and you will be keeping fly breeding delectables from your trash can and kitchen.

④ This might seem really obvious, but put food in the fridge. SO, of course certain types of fruits and veggies prefer to be at room temperature, but most everything can stand to be kept in the fridge, and away from the clutches of the tiny flying beast!

Those steps taken, YOU ARE READY TO BEGIN A MORE AGGRESSIVE APPROACH. FRUIT FLIES ARE FAIRLY DUMB. THAT BEING SAID, THERE ARE A NUMBER OF WAYS TO CREATIVELY TRICK ONE.

① IF you don't want to deal with catching the flies yourself, you can try a predacious plant. You can turn your animosity towards the fly into life-giving food to a curious looking plant. We have two Venus Fly Traps, one Cobra Lily, and one Purple Pitcher. There are also sundew Plants available. All of these plants digest a trapped fly as a source of food although their methods differ. I find that ours do little in the way of reducing our fly problem because they are usually covered to control their humidity and flies can't get to them. They're pretty cool looking though! I give them a 1-Fly Rating —

FEED ME

② Once, we set out a bowl of fruit and waited for the flies to settle on it. Then we got out our trusty vacuum cleaner (with a hose attachment) and simply sucked them up. You can literally suck them right out of the air. It was sort of fun. After you've collected the flies in the vacuum, you can take the vacuum outside, open the filter, and let the flies go. 3 FLIES!

③ There are a variety of sweet liquid/soap traps you can make. I set out a container filled with ¼ cup vinegar and a drop of liquid dishsoap next to a fly-ridden area. The flies are attracted to vinegar — and the soap in the solution traps them. This trap only caught a few. I GIVE IT A ONE.

④ Similar to number 3, mix 1 cup water with a Tablespoon of sugar and a Tablespoon of white vinegar and a drop of liquid dishsoap in a wide bowl. This trap works, but not really well.

⑤ FRUIT FLIES like Beer as much as we do. I put a dish of beer with a couple of drops of dishsoap in it on our pantry shelf and caught at least a dozen little buggers. I think they got too hammered to fly away! 2 FLIES!

⑥ Lay an almost empty bottle of some sweet alcoholic beverage (liqueur, Guiness, wine) on its side. The bottle should have a long, thin neck. The idea here is that the flies will go in but are too stupid to fly out. I found that my flies were too stupid to fly in and mostly just hung out on the lip of the bottle. a half a fly rating —

⑦ This trap is the coolest to study and by far the most effective. First you get a tall cup or jar. Put some overripe fruit in it (Bananas are good, so is jelly). sprinkle yeast over the fruit. The yeast will help the fruit ferment and smell good to the flies. Then, using paper and tape, fashion a funnel with a mouth as big as the mouth of the jar and an opening just bigger than a fly. Tape the funnel onto the jar, with the small opening on the inside. You'll be amazed how quickly this trap fills. Then you can untape the funnel outside and let them go. (or keep them and watch them make babies). FOUR FLY RATING!

for females that don't know shit about cars but want to

About 8 months ago, I took my car to Midas for their "summer trip check special." For around $30 they checked everything on my car that could possibly need work before a long trip. They told me I needed new brake pads and removal of glaze on the brake disk. Cost: $190. For the first time ever I chose to trust my instincts instead of allowing the mechanic to take me for a chump because I'm a girl. I told him I would take care of it and he tried to convince me it needed to be fixed immediately. I told him thanks, then with a little help and advice I fixed the brakes my damn self. Cost: $23. That was my first big lesson on DIY mechanics. I had had my '96 Hyuandai Accent for about 6 months at the time. Someday I'll have a hot pink or metallic red hot rod with lots of chrome, but for now this is what I can afford. It's the first car I've ever had that wasn't crap and I've decided if I'm going to own a good car, I need to learn how to take care of it. In the year I've had this car, I've learned some basic maintenance and repair stuff that I know will save you time, stress, and hopefully lots and lots of money.

Maintenance/Repair Manuals

The Haynes Repair Manual ($10-$15 at most auto parts stores. If car is more than 20-30 yrs.old, you may have to order) and the Owner's Manual that comes with your car (if the former owner still has it) are your first necessities. These will be your textbooks. Read your owner's manual thoroughly and skim the Haynes manual. Compare diagrams and photos with what's under your hood. Try and identify as many pieces and parts as you can. Keep them both in your car.

Your Fluids

They are the first things you should get to know under the hood. Using your manuals, find all of them. The basics are: oil, windshield washer, brake, engine coolant/antifreeze and power steering. They should be labeled and easy to find. Check all of them once a week during normal use. The level should always be between the min. and max.lines. You can buy all of these fluids at any auto parts store, Target, even 7-11. Store them in your trunk because they usually sell in more than one use quantities.

###

Oil

A) Checking it
Oil is so important it needs it's own category. If your car ever runs out of oil, your engine will lock up. An engine cannot be unlocked, so either you buy a new engine or scrap the car. Be obsessive about maintaining your oil! Checking the oil is part of that. It's a little more work than checking the other fluids. Locate your dipstick, it shouldn't be too far from your engine oil filler cap. Remove it, wipe clean with a paper towel, reinsert it, withdraw it, and make sure it falls between the min. and max. marks. If lower than min., add oil immediately. Look at the pavement under your car for any fresh oil. You could have a leak. If you do, you must go to a pesky

mechanic immediately.
B) Changing it
Change your oil every 3000-5000 miles. Your car will be happier and live longer. "Changing" the oil means draining the old oil out and replacing it with new. Wear clothes that you don't mind ruining. Never mess with oil when the engine is hot and never never start your car without oil in it! (I did that once)

You'll need:
1) 3-5 quarts of oil--depending on size of engine. Use SAE 10W-30 or 10W-40 for normal driving conditions.
2) An oil filter--must fit your specific car, tell guy at auto parts store your year, make, and model and the filter will magically appear.
3) Wrench--to fit your drain plug. This is where the old oil drains.
4) Large shallow pan--to catch the oil. Look in garden depts. of hardware stores.
5) Funnel
6) And if you're miss priss, Work gloves and rag

Here's a brief overview of what you'll do. Read your owners manual or ask for more details if you need them. I suggest someone who knows what they're doing to oversee you the first time you do this.
1) set the parking brake
2) open hood, remove oil filter cap
3) slide under car, make sure pan is under drain plug
4) use wrench to turn drain plug counterclockwise, remove it and move fast or you'll have a hand full of oil.
5) When oil stops draining, replace drain plug.
6) Make sure pan is under oil filter, remove it by unscrewing with your hands. If too tight, you'll need an oil filter wrench or stronger hands.
7) Install new filter. Follow directions on box. Make sure the old gasket (round, black plastic piece resembling a washer) comes off.
8) Add oil
9) Use funnel to pour drained oil from pan into empty bottles the new oil came in.
10) recycle old oil at auto parts store.
11) According to Central Virginia Waste Management, the bottles themselves can't be recycled because the petroleum is too difficult to rinse.

I Don't Drive Without

car jack (good one around $50)
tire iron
spare tire/doughnut
various wrenches (socket set even better)
at least 1 quart oil
medium bottle water (for radiator if car overheats)
jumper cables (booster pack even better. You can jump start without another car)

Random money, time, & Potentially Life Saving Tips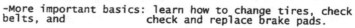

-More important basics: learn how to change tires, check belts, and   check and replace brake pads.

–Buy the LOWEST octane/cheapest gas. Higher octane gases are formulated for high performance engines only.

–Scope out nice apartment complexes for community garden hoses. (There's one at Three Chopt West Apts.) Bring bucket, sponge, cleaner and you've got a free car wash.

–"Goo-Gone", sold with cleaners, will remove tar and black streaks.

–If you have scratches on your car's body, especially if they've begun to rust, you can buy little containers of primer and touch-up paint at auto parts store.

–Get lots of help. Always ask questions and get advice at any opportunity to talk to someone who knows more about cars than you.

–Don't pull off onto the side of the interstate by yourself unless your car will not move. I don't even pull over for cops unless I'm in a well lit area. Fuck 'em. If I don't feel safe, I'm not pulling over the second they flash a blue light. Trust your gut instinct.

If you've been wanting to learn about your car but didn't know where to start, I hope this helps. A car is an intimidating machine and this is only a start. You will be in a constant state of learning when you start caring for your car. It takes energy and patience. And don't assume that every guy knows exactly what he's doing under the hood because he's a guy. They could be clueless, but are usually pretty willing to spend hours connecting wires in the dark, freeze their asses off, squeeze into tiny, grimy garages, break tools, get filthy, and push your car across busy intersections, determined to come to our rescue. This is great. The only problem is that we are usually more than willing to let them. So let them, but pay attention, observe them, ask questions and you might be learning something together. Most likely you do have a cousin, uncle, brother, dad, friend, boyfriend, husband, or grandfather that knows more about cars than you. Think of them as a resource, it can only help.

While you're learning how to care for your crappy, cheap, generic, yuppie or stupid car, dream about restoring your own customized '56 cherry red Chevy Bel Air with matching interior, or a silvery pink two-toned 1930 chopped Ford Coupe, or a 1932 convertible roadster or. . .

FIX YER BIKE!!!

Recently I started coordinating a DIY section for an online zine. The idea is to have a resource where people can go to find out how to do the stuff they want to do Silk Screening, Gardening, Repairs (Bike, Home, Musical Instruments, etc.) So we've been inviting anybody who knows how to do something to get involved, and write for it. If your interested, write me or check out the DIY section on Misterridiculous.com. Following is a piece I wrote for that. With all my ranting about bicycles, I thought a little fixer upper DIY might be helpful.

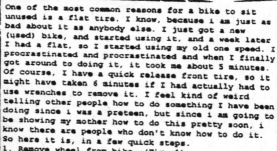

One of the most common reasons for a bike to sit unused is a flat tire. I know, because i am just as bad about it as anybody else. I just got a new (used) bike, and started using it, and a week later I had a flat, so I started using my old one speed. I procrastinated and procrastinated and when I finally got around to doing it, it took me about 5 minutes. Of course, I have a quick release front tire, so it might have taken 6 minutes if I had actually had to use wrenches to remove it. I feel kind of weird telling other people how to do something I have been doing since i was a preteen, but since i am going to be showing my mother how to do this pretty soon, i know there are people who don't know how to do it. So here it is, in a few quick steps.

1. Remove wheel from bike. (Fig. 1)
2. Let all the air out of the tire. (if you have a valve core remover, that
works really well!)
3. Slip a tire lever, or screwdriver between the tire and the rim and pry edge of wheel over rim. It's best to use a dull one so that you don't poke new holes in the tube. (Fig. 2)
4. Continue around the tire doing the same thing until you have one entire edge of the tire off.
5. Push the valve stem into the tire, reach under to pull it out the rest of the way, and then pull the whole tube out, being careful to leave in the fabric or rubber rim strip. This protects your tube from the ends of the spokes.
6. At this point you have a couple options; you can either spend $2.50-$5 and just throw a new tube in, or you can spend 99 cents and patch the tire. Patching the tire doesn't take that long, and I personally would go that route. If you're going to just replace the tube, skip to step 14
7. Unless you can tell where the leak is, fill the tube with air. Sometimes you will be able to tell where the leak is just by the escape of air. If you can't, fill up a sink with water and immerse the tube a section at a time, working around the tube until you see bubbles. Sometimes the leak will be very slow, and it will take a bit more looking because you'll only get a bubble every few seconds. Pay special attention to the valve stem. Sometimes a loose core can be the only problem. (Fig. 3)

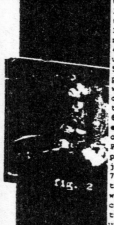

fig. 2

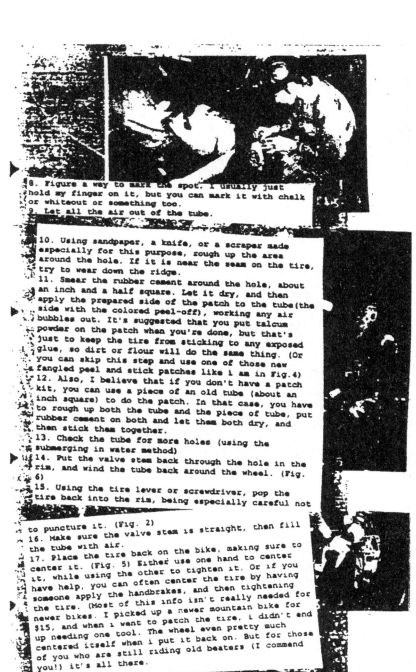

8. Figure a way to mark the spot. I usually just hold my finger on it, but you can mark it with chalk or whiteout or something too.

9. Let all the air out of the tube.

10. Using sandpaper, a knife, or a scraper made especially for this purpose, rough up the area around the hole. If it is near the seam on the tire, try to wear down the ridge.

11. Smear the rubber cement around the hole, about an inch and a half square. Let it dry, and then apply the prepared side of the patch to the tube (the side with the colored peel-off), working any air bubbles out. It's suggested that you put talcum powder on the patch when you're done, but that's just to keep the tire from sticking to any exposed glue, so dirt or flour will do the same thing. (Or you can skip this step and use one of those new fangled peel and stick patches like i am in Fig.4)

12. Also, I believe that if you don't have a patch kit, you can use a piece of an old tube (about an inch square) to do the patch. In that case, you have to rough up both the tube and the piece of tube, put rubber cement on both and let them both dry, and then stick them together.

13. Check the tube for more holes (using the submerging in water method)

14. Put the valve stem back through the hole in the rim, and wind the tube back around the wheel. (Fig. 6)

15. Using the tire lever or screwdriver, pop the tire back into the rim, being especially careful not to puncture it. (Fig. 2)

16. Make sure the valve stem is straight, then fill the tube with air.

17. Place the tire back on the bike, making sure to center it. (Fig. 5) Either use one hand to center it, while using the other to tighten it. Or if you have help, you can often center the tire by having someone apply the handbrakes, and then tightening the tire. (Most of this info isn't really needed for newer bikes. I picked up a newer mountain bike for $15, and when i went to patch the tire, i didn't end up needing one tool. The wheel even pretty much centered itself when i put it back on. But for those of you who are still riding old beaters (I command you!) it's all there.

STOPPING FLATS

Are you tired of punctured tires and constantly patching flats? Then puncture-proof your tires! Here's how:

Take and old inner tube that's past its prime (ya know, 10 or more patches) and cut through it (fig a). Then cut it down the center so it's just a flat piece of rubber (fig b).

FIG A

FIG B

Then cut the rubber into three-inch pieces. Make the width skinny enough so that the pieces fit along the inside of the tire wall, but fat enough so that it covers the area of the tire that touches the ground.

Take these pieces and glue them to the inside of your tire. To glue them in, you can use anything that will do the job of sticking them to the tire. The pressure of the inflated tube will keep them in place, so the glue only needs to hold them in place until you get the tube in.

This gives you an extra layer of rubber to stop destructive objects and greatly reduces your risk of a flat. The tire on my chopper is almost down to the wire, but with this advanced technology, I haven't gotten a flat yet. I learned this from some people at Spurkraft in Portland.

BiKE TiP

IF YOUR SEATPOST IS JUST A LITTLE TOO SMALL,
AND WON'T TIGHTEN ALL THE WAY, YOU
CAN MAKE A SHIM FROM A SODA CAN. JUST
USE A SCISSORS TO CUT THE ENDS OFF A
CAN

THEN YOU ROLL THE TIN SMALL ENOUGH to
SLIP INTO YOUR SEAT TUBE. I ALSO CUT
A LITTLE EXTRA OFF SO IT WAS ABOUT 2-3
inches tall. THEN YOU JUST SLIP ABOUT
HALF OF IT INTO THE SEAT TUBE

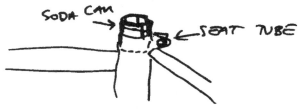

SODA CAN → ← SEAT TUBE

THEN YOU JUST PUT YOUR SEAT POST
IN THAT, push it down & tighten it up.
(the tin won't usually push all the way
m. on mine, ABout ¼-½" stayed ABOVE
THE SEATpost. this is good in Case you
need to Remove it Sometime

THANX TO the Guy AT Freewheel who told me this
INSTEAD OF TAKING MY $12.00

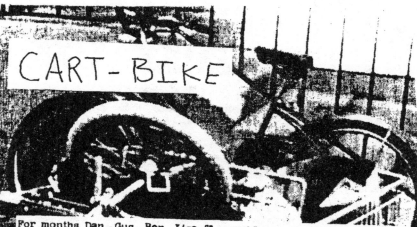

CART-BIKE

For months Dan, Gus, Ben, Lisa & myself have been talking about building bicycles. I've mentioned before about me & Ben's obsession with High Wheeler/Penny Farthing bikes. But neither of us knew how to weld, and we were having trouble figuring out all the details. So gradually, our focus shifted towards more utilitarian bicycles. Mostly pickup/truck bikes and cart bikes. We still were planning on doing welding though. Two people offered their assistance. Since Gus was as excited about the prospects as we were, it seemed like things would work. One problem still remained. Gus didn't have equipment, and the equipment at the community house where Dan lives was frozen in the garage. (The garage door couldn't be moved for at least a month due to inches of ice around it) And we didn't even know if we had the right equipment, because the only person who ever used it was gone for 5 months or more.

But when I ran across plans for a bicycle cart with no need for welding, ideas started churning. I didn't like the plans, and they were kind of incomplete besides. But the basic idea that I latched onto was the use of U-clamps. A lot could be accomplished with those little wonders. The plans I found (they were either in Seedhead, Luddite Tech Zine or How 2 Zine.) suggested U-clamping forks to the side of a cart. We thought they'd move around too much and decided to try an axle (still using u-clamps to attach everything.) Their plans also called for some weird bent pipe contraption for steering. We decided to clamp the forks directly to the cart. This of course was all before we even had a cart in our possession. So it was all just speculation. Then we got our hands on some carts & Monday, got together for our first building session.

Gus towed a cart I'd left in Ben's backyard over to my garage where we had plenty of parts and tools. We set about to finding pieces to put it together. We wanted a girls frame, so it'd be easy to get on and off. I didn't have many, but we found a nice yellow one with no wheels or handlebars (or neck.) We found a back wheel and a couple front ones and started piecing it together It was about 4 hours that night, and mostly we just learned what wouldn't work. The allthread axle wasn't the same thread as bicycle axles, so we had to jerry-rig it. I'll save you the boring details of how that worked, because it ended up that the axle was too flimsy anyway. We tried to clamp the forks to the cart & had trouble there too. First we clamped it too low so that the pedals hit the ground, and we didn't clamp it to main braces, so it broke the little welds on the cart. We had a brain storming session and put the parts away for the night.

I had to work the next day, so I gave Ben the key to the garage and showed him where the tools were. When I got home, they were putting the finishing touches on the basic design. I'll give details on it's assembly later. We took it for a test drive, and it was hella hard to drive! Wow! It took muscle to steer, and if you steered too sharp, it would tip over. And when you started to steer, it would pull even harder in that direction, so that you had to hold it back. At this point it had no brakes or gears. We had Lisa sit in it, since she was smallest. With a load, it was much easier to drive. We each took turns in it, and even with 165 pounds, it held up and drove fine. So then we brought it back to the garage and put a neck on it, which we clamped to the grocery cart for extra support and to attach the gear shifters to. (You should definitely have some gears on a cart bike.) We hooked up a back brake, which was also attached to the handle.

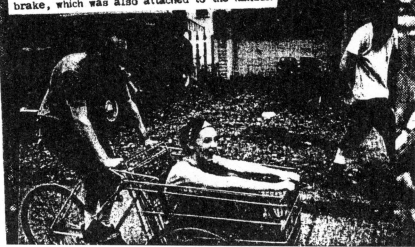

Okay, the first thing you're going to have to do is get your hands on a cart. Metal ones are the only ones worth grabbing. I say, grab the biggest one you can find (but then I've never tried a small one.) Once you have that, you just grab yourself a hacksaw, and cut the basket off the bottom half of the cart. Just cut the four legs as close as you can to the basket. We also

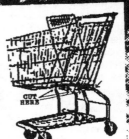

CUT HERE

took the plastic handle off the cart, so that whoever originally owned the cart wouldn't come after us trying to get it back. Take off any identifying marks, even if you dumpstered the thing. (rather than finding it on the side of the road or in a vacant lot or something.)

Next you're going to need an adult sized bike to attach the cart to. I would highly suggest a women's bike, since they're much easier to get on and off of. I would also highly suggest that it be a 10 speed, since you'll be happy to have the extra gears when you're trying to pedal a basket full of groceries (or bricks, or people, or whatever) uphill.

Here's a list of other things you'll need to complete this project:

- 6 or more small U-clamps (about an inch across)
- 1 large U-clamp (big enough to fit around the head tube of your bike)
- 2 matching front wheels & coinciding forks. (I would suggest at least 26inch wheels)
- 2-4 hose clamps
- 1 tin can

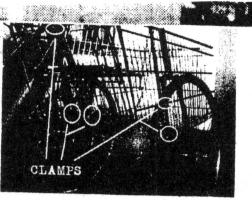

CLAMPS

Take the forks and wheels and position them on the sides of the cart. You can screw around with this and try to figure out where they work best, but we found that the forks should stick past the bottom of the cart a couple inches, and should be pretty close to the back. One reason for this is that most of a cart is composed of weak little bars. If you attach the forks to those, the little welds will break, and it won't be very strong. There are only a few strong bars that forks should be attached to. We chose a point near the back where some of the main supports are. Two of these strong bars crossed each other, and we put the U-clamps there. Put the U-clamps on, and tighten them down a bit. Make sure the cart sits level, and then tighten everything up. (I've darkened up the strong bars, so they're more visible in the picture. Notice the clamps (circled in white) are all attached to at least one of these.).

Now, pull the front wheel off your bike. Remove the front brake, and both the brake handles. Now spread open the neck and remove your handlebars. (You'll want to leave the neck, as you'll be using it later. Also, using the handlebars to spread the neck open will make the job easier later on.)

We tried to file the dropouts on the fork wide enough to accept the bar that runs across the bottom of the back of the basket, but gave up as we were in such a hurry to get the thing done. It evidently didn't need to be done, but I think it might be a good idea anyway. So then you just turn the forks around, so they're backwards and center them on the bar that runs across the bottom of the back of the cart. Use a U-clamp on each side of the fork near the bottom to attach it to a strong part of the back of the cart. Then use your big U-clamp to attach the neck to the back part of the cart. To make the attachment just a little more secure, we spread open the neck, and twisted the two pieces of the handle with a channel locks so they would slide into it, then tightened it up. To get a really tight fit, we would have needed some old tubing or tin can strips or something, but we left it as is. We also attached our gear shifters to the neck. Because the backs of most carts flap open, you'll need to use a few hose clamps to hold it shut. We put a couple on the bottom, and a couple on the sides.

hose clamps

Now you've kind of got a choice with the brakes. You can just leave off the front one, and attach the back handle to the cart like we did. Or you can put brakes on both the forks attached to the cart, and have them up in front where all the stopping power is. This is what I would have done, but the bike I was using didn't have any brakes, and I had trouble scrounging up even one. This is where that tin can will come in handy. You'll have to cut strips of it to wrap around the cart handle, so you can tightly attach the brake handles. In the pictures, it looks like we duct taped ours on, but that's just there to cover the edges of the tin can. Some grips would make the handle a bit more comfortable. (maybe some of those foam 10 speed ones or something)

I haven't gone into every single detail about putting one of these together, because every single bike/cart combination is going to be different. With each you'll encounter your own special brand of problems along the way. If you've never worked on a bike before, this might not be the project for you. Probably learning to adjust your brakes & gears, and change your tires is a good place to start. If you've done some work on bikes, this should come pretty easy for you. The hardest part for us was coming up with the basic design, and doing it without any welds. We've fixed that problem for you. Now go to it!

Just to let you know, our concern about the forks moving was well founded. Our forks do move a bit, but if the bike is moving forward, and especially with a load, the problem is self-correcting. It has yet to be a real problem. These things are pretty difficult to drive. I found that it's much easier to steer by leaning, than by trying to turn the cart. The problem is that you have to shift your weight the opposite of the way you want to go. It's sort of difficult to explain, but once you have yours built, you'll see what I mean. It's definitely not built for speed. In order to keep control, you have to move sort of slow. It's good for getting loads of stuff (like groceries) but I wouldn't want to use it as an every day bike (unless I was hauling a lot of stuff every day, and then I would build a trailer.)

By the way, if you come up with any fabulous variations (that don't require welding) on this design, write and let us know about them, and we'll pass the info along.

matte resist

REFLEX is to get pissed off. To talk shit. To get drunk. To bicker and complain. It's so standard I see it in the suits and ties. You can even catch them spitting bullets about rules and regulations when the leash gets too tight, about bureaucracy when it's confusing and ineffectual (which it surely always is), about crooked cops when they happened to beat the wrong person within an inch of their life, about homelessness when it invades their neighborhood or occupies a childs' life, about minimum-wage when it's a single-mother who really believes in the American Dream, about education when it means their own teenaged kids hardly have a third-grade knowledge of historical events. It's so fucking normal. Reflex is there. It has to be there. Even my own parents have reflexes sometimes. It is important and essential to get pissed, to get outraged. At very least it is important to have any sort of reflex at all. If you don't have an opinion you're as good as dead. If you can't exhale you can't inhale. Reflex happens because it has to. If it didn't happen we'd know that our bodies are no longer our own, that we're not made of flesh and bone but of bolts and metal.

REACTION is throwing bricks. It's riots in the streets and bombs in the Capitol Building. It's Molotov Cocktails. It's stealing food and eating out of dumpsters. It's fighting back. It's picketing, striking, and marching. It is petitions and court cases. It can range from asking for permission to demanding solutions. It means working with the system. It means compromise. It's a defense. It's important and essential. It's saying "NO!"

ACTION is growing vegetables, squatting or building houses, occupying factories, and making clothing. Action is saying "yes" to community needs. It is saying "YES" to whatever we want. It is making networks of skilled laborers and service-people. It is drawing up our own plan. It is building our own future. It is important and essential.

PUNK ROCK IS REFLEX.
THROWING ROCKS IS REACTION.
BUILDING COMMUNITY IS ACTION!

I have spent the last 6 or 7 years handing out pamphlets, holding up signs on street corners, whining and complaining, and throwing bricks through windows and slashing tires. I've spent so much time in dumpsters, lecture halls, meetings, gardens, and books. So much time that it is what I'm referred to as... an activist. That's what I do, I am an activist. And most likely most of you who are reading this are too. But it depends upon how we define the word "activist". I believe that it is defined quite loosely. That if you take part in any sort of rebellion besides simple Reflex it is "Action". And Action is done by activists, I guess.

But the term "activism" is defined loosely. The larger portion of activism is actually Reaction. The non-corporate press is important, not only because it is non-corporate but because it is a press. Pressing the news and views of the community is essential. It is important for us to know how others feel and to have conflict. It is important to know what is going on in our community. And that's why the press is important. It is actively taking part, and allowing our voices to be heard. The press is Action. But the larger chunk of "activism" is actually Reaction. It is finding out about injustices and speaking out about them (ie: marching in the streets for justice for Mumia Abu-Jamal or to end the sanctions in Iraq, etc.). It is reacting to an injustice that is happening. And although it is essential to do so, it is reactionary. So the term "activist" encompasses action and reaction.

Reaction can be draining. It's an uphill battle. It's constantly saying "no." It is necessary but due to its nature it can be depressing. It can also distract our view of where we really want to be heading instead of just constantly worrying about where we don't want to be. Just because we're not where we don't want to be doesn't mean we're where we want to be.

To be involved with action is to make your own rules.

This in no way at all is to demean reactionary activism. I have found that there needs to be a balance with the two to prevent burnout, depression, or to become jaded. Reaction is vital and I continue to take part in those struggles. But it is important to take part in action that is positive also. I believe in activism that says "yes". "This is not our list of demands. This is what we're going to do," and then to do them.

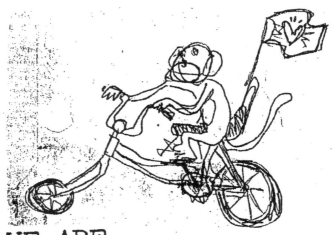

WE ARE

Where others might say, "we'll just make
do," we shout, "All this and more, too!"
Broken bicycles and half-rotted vegetables,
scrap wood, some duct tape, free rides and
DIY. In our day-to-day lives, we are an
entire network of resources and resource-
fulness. We are scrappers and scavengers,
sleuths, lockpicks and scam artists; not to
mention self-taught mechanics, historians,
weavers, artists, explorers, gardeners,
farmers and writers; inventors and broad-
casters and publishers, boat-builders and
religious scholars and all-around fixer-
uppers; carpenters, electricians, pirates
and folklorists, anthropologists, archivists
and teachers; propagandists, agitators,
musicians, librarians, cultural dilettantes,
community voices; students, learners, econo-
mists, mapmakers, printers, herbalists,
activists, engineers, chefs, tailors,
parents and alchemists; all this and more.

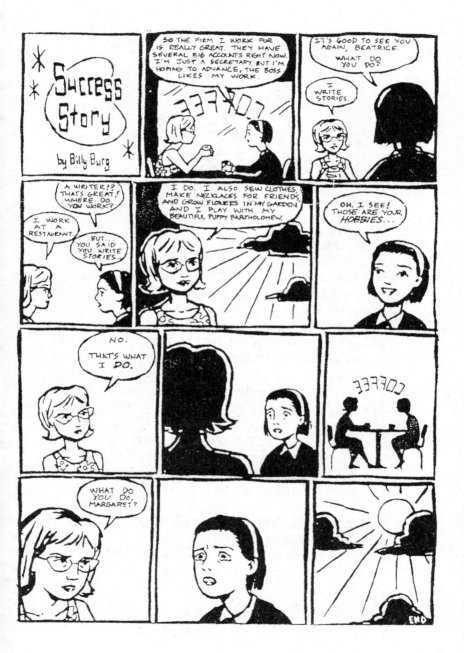

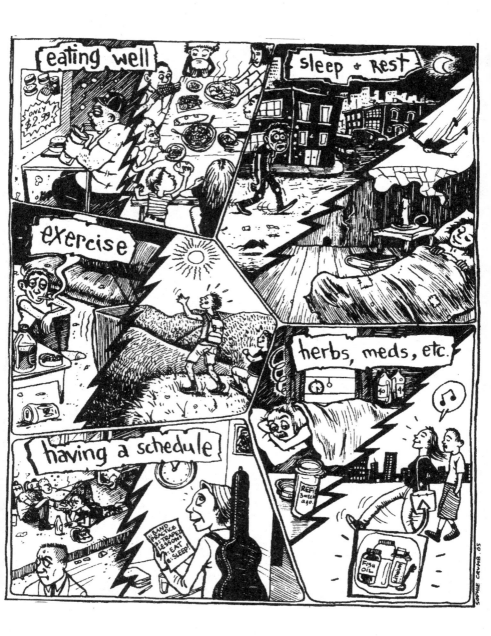

INDEX

- - - - - - -

FOR FURTHER READING ON:

Change your life and the world around you.

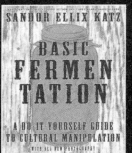
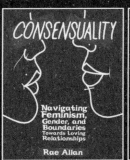
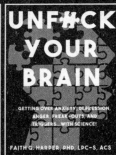
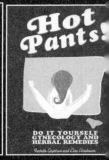
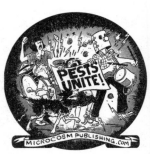
Read more about the DIY Revolution:

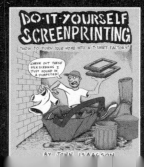
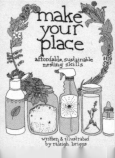
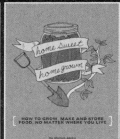
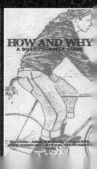